Positive Smear

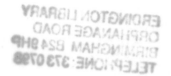
Susan Quilliam

Foreword by Dame Josephine Barnes, President of the Women's Nationwide Cancer Control Campaign

This second edition published in 1992
by Charles Letts & Co Ltd
Letts of London House
Parkgate Road
London SW11 4NQ

First published in 1989
by Penguin Books
27 Wright's Lane
London W8 5TZ

© Susan Quilliam 1992
Susan Quilliam has asserted her moral right to be identified as the author of this work

Photographs supplied by the National Medical Slide Bank (Figs 7, 8 and 9) and the
Science Photo Library (Figs 1 and 2)
Illustrations by Tek Art
Cover and book style design by Sotomayor Designers Ltd
Cover photography by Adri Berger

ISBN 1 85238 366 6

A CIP catalogue record for this book is available from the British Library

'Letts' is a registered trademark of Charles Letts & Co Limited

Printed and bound in Great Britain

Contents

Acknowledgements

In preparing the acknowledgement list for a book of this kind, to which many
people have contributed time, energy and skill, there is always the fear that
someone has been left out. So I would like to begin with a thank-you to
everybody who helped me, both in the original writing of the book, the
intervening conferences and 'word-spreading', and in this relaunch,
whether or not their name is mentioned!

I should like to thank all the women who were willing to share their
experiences and emotions with me, both those named below and those who
preferred not to be named, as well as their friends and families.
Alain Allard, Amy Redfield, Andrew Woolley, Catherine O'Neill, Cedric,
Diana, Dorothy Newton, Elizabeth Butters, Emma Allard, Evelyn Marsden,
Frances, Heather Robinson, Hilda, Ian, Jan Hardy, Jane, Jane Ginsborg,
Janet Wild (RGN), Janice, Joanne Hailey, Judith Roche, Julia Tozer, Julie,
Lily Hopkins, Pat Kirwan, Rachel Woolley, Sue Linge, Sue Robaczynski,
Viki Mills, Vivienne Wall.

My thanks to these people and organizations for giving me their specialist
advice and support:
Dr Mary Buchanan, Penny Craddock and all those at the Women's
Nationwide Cancer Control Campaign; Abnormal Smear Care Group of
the Long Eaton and District Volunteer Bureau; Mr Christopher
Balogun-Lynch and Maureen Pruskin of the Myrtle Peach Trust; Toni
Belfield and Jane Urwin of the Family Planning Association; Penny Brohn
and Cynthia Slade, Bristol Cancer Help Centre; Eleanor Brown; Alice
Burns; D Byrne, St Thomas's Hospital; M Saveria Campo, the Beatson
Institute of Cancer Research; Alison Carmichael, Institute of Oncology,
Marie Curie Cancer Care; Professor Dulcie Coleman, St Mary's Hospital;
Ann Cowper; Sian Davies, Marie Curie Cancer Care; Ingrid Docherty, St
Thomas's Hospital; Dr Ian D Duncan, Ninewells Hospital; Jane
Faulkwhynes; Annabel Geddes, Women Against Cervical Cancer; Trish
Goode, Cancer Relief Macmillan Fund; The Gynaecological Nursing
Forum of the Royal College of Nursing; Sally Haslett, St Thomas's
Hospital; Victoria Holt; Lily Hopkins; Pat Iveson, CYNANA; Amanda
Kelsey and Maxine Rosenfield, Cancerlink; Mr Kenney, St Thomas's

Positive Smear

Hospital; Dr Pat Last and Geraldine O'Connor, BUPA; June Macpherson of Marie Stopes House; Sr Gill Marsh and Vivienne Wall, The United Kingdom Association of Colposcopy Nurses; Dr Ann McPherson; Dr A J Robertson, Perth Royal Infirmary; Anthony C Silverstone, Consultant Gynaecologist, University College Hospital; Andrew Sincock, University College London; Elizabeth Skinner, Cancer Research Campaign; Donald Stevens and Colin Ryder-Richardson, New Approaches to Cancer; Yvonne Terry and Nikki Hill, BACUP; the Health Editors of Time Out and City Limits; Dr Michael Turner, Coombe Lying-in Hospital; Trish Vezgoff, University of Wollongong; Susan Williams; Dr Jan de Winter, Emeritus Senior Consultant in Radiotherapy and Oncology, Royal Sussex County Hospital Brighton, Founder Director of the Clinic for Cancer Prevention Advice Brighton; Patricia Wejr and all the staff at Women's Health (formerly The Women's Health and Reproductive Rights Information Centre); Glenis Burgess, Mary Cooper, Nancy McKeith of Yorkshire Women's Video; Sue Mack, Lisa Saffron, Monika Schwartz and all the many women who helped to make the *Positive Smear – Positive Approach Conference* and *Update Day* so successful.

Thanks go too to Dr Penny Ward for proofing the original manuscript, and Dr Carmel Coulter for providing the original introduction; Cynthia Alves, Pam Dix and Jenny Condie for their work on the original book; Patrick Walker, Consultant Gynaecologist, The Royal Free Hospital for his time and inspiration, Barbara Levy, Vikki Matten, Felicity Sinclair, Jenni Tibble, Cortina Butler, Penny Simpson and everyone else at Letts who has worked on the book, for their inspiration and work on this edition. I should like to thank especially June MacPherson of Marie Stopes House for her instant reaction to my requests for help; Anne Szareweski for her delightful, unstinting and unselfish co-operation in this project, and my husband Ian for his unfailing love and support. A final acknowledgement is due to Mr Albert Singer and the staff of the Royal Northern Hospital for treating me when I had a positive smear diagnosed, and for their very particular contribution in motivating me to write this book.

Foreword

It is a pleasure to welcome this new and revised edition of a book which has proved an invaluable resource to women, their partners and families and to medical professionals.

The author, Susan Quilliam, bases the opening chapter on her personal reaction of fear and dismay on getting the news that she has had a 'positive smear'. She felt a desperate need for information, counselling and reassurance and it was this that motivated her to write this book. It covers in detail and in simple, easily understood language what any woman may expect if she gets such a report. This includes the various examinations and treatments that may be recommended.

Perhaps the most important message of this book is that a positive smear is not a sentence of death and does not necessarily indicate cancer.

Excellent advice is given on what to expect when visiting a family doctor or hospital clinic. In each case there is a list of questions to ask. The process of biopsy and the various methods of cauterization are described, with the after effects to be expected – incidentally often minimized by medical and nursing staff. The processes of hospital admission and operation are also described.

Sadly, communication with the professionals is not always all it might be. Medical and nursing staff are often too overworked to give the best investigation and treatment to too many patients. Medical and nursing students have to be taught and most patients will be pleased to co-operate if the needs are properly explained and the patient is not submitted to indignities.

The importance of good general health is stressed. There is a useful discussion of contraception and of the possible anxieties and problems of the male partner. Many may feel a sense of guilt in particular about sexual relations. Here counselling and understanding, and not a censorious attitude, are essential.

This book is very much in sympathy with the aims of the Women's Nationwide Cancer Control Campaign. It was founded in 1965 by a group of women deeply concerned at the number of women dying from cancer of the cervix. There has been great progress since then and the majority of women at risk in the United Kingdom is now being screened. The deaths that do occur are mainly in those women who have never had a smear test. In 1989, WNCCC established a telephone Helpline to provide counselling, information and emotional support.

Susan Quilliam rightly emphasizes the fact that a positive smear is not always a disaster. It may provide an opportunity for the woman concerned, and her partner, to reassess her life style and to enjoy better health in the future.

The Women's Nationwide Cancer Control Campaign continues its work in cancer prevention and health education., This book explains to women and to the professionals who care for them how these aims may be best achieved.

July 1992
Dame Josephine Barnes DBE, DM, FRCP, FRCS, FRCOG
President of the Women's Nationwide Cancer Control Campaign

First words

‘ When a woman has a positive smear, she faces issues around her sexuality, her fertility and her mortality. ’
(Dr. P.W.)

On 19 December 1981, my world fell apart. Sitting on the steps of my flat, I read and reread the slip of paper from my doctor that informed me that I had a 'positive smear', and that I needed to come and see him as a matter of urgency. I had no idea what this meant. I knew that I had had a routine cervical smear a few weeks ago, and had been expecting the result. I knew that both my parents had died of cancer. And I also knew that my doctor, a placid and reassuring man, had used the word 'urgent' in his letter. I am, I think, an intelligent woman, possessed of a normal amount of resourcefulness and ability. But faced with that small slip of paper, I broke down and sobbed uncontrollably.

What happened to me then was fairly typical of what happens to women after they have had a positive smear. I went 'urgently' to my doctor, who referred me for further

1

examination. I saw a consultant, who assured me that my condition was minor – and then wrote to me a week or two later saying that he had been mistaken. I did need treatment; I had an advanced form of pre-cancer.

My reactions were very mixed: I sometimes felt an inner conviction that what they had found was not pre-cancer but cancer, and that I was going to die. Often I found myself remembering that this was an illness of the cervix; how would it affect my sex life? What about having children? I felt particularly powerless when faced with medical professionals, strangely vulnerable to them because the condition I had was sexual in nature.

A month later, having gone in to hospital once and been sent home again because I had a cold, I received my treatment. They used diathermy, a cauterization method that involved a general anaesthetic and left me for a week afterwards both sore and tired, and with bouts of nausea caused by the post-operation antibiotics.

My check-up pronounced me cured. One morning, a few months after the operation, I woke to find that I was feeling suddenly and inexplicably well, in a way that I hadn't done for years. I have had normal, negative smears ever since.

But that was not the end of it. I was, even at the time, taken aback by the strength of my reaction to what all the facts told me was a fairly minor medical problem. I was sometimes frightened that I would die, embarrassed that I had an illness in a sexual area, angry that it had happened to me. I had to stop and take stock of where I was, think through my life, my relationships, whether I wanted children. I had, more than at any time in my past, to fight for what I needed, medically and emotionally.

2

When the time came to write a book about having a positive smear, I took my own experience as a starting point. I wanted to know if other women had felt the same as I did – sometimes coping well, but sometimes confused and negative about the whole process. Had they asked the same questions I had about whether they would live, bear children, regain their sexuality? What sort of things did women need; what had I needed, all those years ago, to help me cope – and more than cope – with what was happening?

I took a deep breath and began asking questions, of doctors, nurses, friends, partners – but above all, of the women themselves. I did over fifty interviews and took even more written evidence. ·The answers I got amazed me; a positive smear was, as one woman put it, 'far more than a cut on your arm'. Not all women felt like this. Some had regarded it as a mere ripple in their lives. But many had been concerned about the whole experience, many had had to stop and think, not just about whether they were free for the next hospital appointment, but about much deeper issues. As I continued, talking not only to patients but also to medical professionals it became clear that the positive smear 'process' as it exists in Britain today is capable of raising questions about many areas in a woman's life.

Having raised them, however, it then fails to give clear-cut answers. The smear test is one of the few tests that can detect cancer in its pre-cancerous stages, when a 100 per cent cure is still possible. What worries many women, however, is the underlying urgency to most approaches to the problem, for the condition, once identified, needs monitoring to avoid the threat of serious illness. To complicate matters further, the cause of cervical cancer or pre-cancer is still debatable. The question of whether it is linked to sexual behaviour is particularly fraught, and in our society a positive smear result can provoke a barrage of value judgements that rebound not only on women but also on their partners. In short, when you have a positive smear, you open a whole Pandora's box of issues.

It seems to me, from the women I have spoken to, that saying such things is not scaremongering: in the first place, a woman who has a positive smear is one of the lucky ones – she has been spotted, and now has an almost 100 per cent chance of complete recovery; secondly, the extraordinary medical advances of recent years mean that women can now survive cervical cancer and the day-to-day medical competence means they are often treated effectively and with respect. So I am not suggesting to women that they sit and worry about what their positive smear result means. For I do not need to suggest this – women are already worrying quite enough.

After a positive smear, a woman faces a whole mixture of medical and emotional challenges, and to admit this is a step forward. For although we deny it, we are caught in a spiral of reassurance and mixed messages which inhibit real action. Only if we accept the fact that we have a problem can we begin to do something about it.

So what should we do? When I spoke to women, the central question I put was this: what do we as women (and those around us) need, in order to make sense of what is happening to us as we go through the positive smear process? And the answer I received was 'information . . . clarity . . . a knowledge of what is going to happen to me . . . a way of coping with my husband . . . a way of coping with myself . . .

someone to tell me it's all right to cry . . . someone to tell me what all the mixed messages mean . . .'

In response to these needs then, a large part of this book deals with the physical aspects of cervical conditions: the biology, the causes, the treatments. But an equally large part of it is about the emotional aspects: how does what is happening affect how you feel about yourself? How does it affect your relationships with other people? How can you take control of what is happening? How can you make decisions about your health and your treatment? What skills and strengths can you develop as you move through the process? And how can you use positively the fact that it may make you stop and question things?

In particular, I have tried to accept that having a positive smear raises lots of questions, and that often there are no easy answers, only further challenges. A woman may not know what has caused her condition – but she can begin to look at where she might be vulnerable. She may have to question her sex life – but she can do this from choice and not because she is being blamed or frightened. She may feel helpless in her dealings with medical professionals – but she may also begin to realize that she has the power to become involved in the process of her own health.

The book, then, is divided into four parts. The section on *Process* takes a step-by-step look at what happens from the moment a positive smear result is received. The *Facts* section gives more 'hard-core' information, both on the biological aspects of the possible conditions a positive smear can indicate, and on the range of possible causes. This section could be read alongside the one on *Process* to gain some understanding of the medical aspects of what is happening. In the section on *Feelings* I have concentrated on the four key issues that women have raised when talking to me, and devoted a chapter to each. The final chapter in this section contains verbatim reports of women's own experiences. At the end of the book is a full *Resource* section of reading matter, people, films and other sources of information and support.

If you have just had a positive smear, use this book where and when appropriate, to guide you through the process. You may not want or need to read every chapter, and may prefer to concentrate on those which are relevant to you at the moment. If you are supporting someone who has just had a positive smear, then read the whole book, to prepare you for what might happen.

If your positive smear has been diagnosed as pre-cancerous, you will find most of the experiences you are likely to have charted in this book, along with the experiences of other women. If your positive smear has been diagnosed as meaning you have cancer, you will perhaps see this book as dealing with only the tip of your particular iceberg. You may want to go on to explore other sources or support groups that address your situation in more detail – and many such organizations are listed in the resource section at the back of this book.

If you have had a positive smear and are now recovered, then read this book to help you assimilate more fully, in retrospect, what happened. And if you have not yet had a positive smear, then remember that in all likelihood someone you know, maybe you yourself, will have one in the not-too-distant future.

If you are a medical professional, please read this book to remind you of what you already know – that it may be a 'minor medical issue, rarely serious' to you, but that for some of us, its discovery means that the world falls apart and needs to be put back together. If you are a medical policy maker, let the book stand as a cry for *more please* – more funds, more staff, more understanding, more attention.

Please also note that I am not a medical professional, despite being qualified in the field of emotional care. So I have not attempted to write a medical work, although all the factual sections of this book are medically sound. My aim has been to gain an understanding of the positive smear experience in a wider context than the purely physical, and to provide a book that complements other, more medically orientated ones.

When I initially wrote these 'First Words', in 1988, I had no idea how far I had succeeded in this aim. Then, my book was somewhat of a voice in the wilderness. But since then, some wonderful things have happened. Firstly, the book was published – an act of faith on the part of the publishing industry. Secondly, other books, articles and studies on the same topic came on the market, adding their weight to the call for the feelings of positive smear patients to be taken seriously. And thirdly, as a result of all this, a group of women and men, patients and professionals alike, came together to explore the issues around the emotional problems of positive smears, in the *Positive Smear – A Positive Approach* Conference. Suddenly, the issues were being aired. Positive smear patients were explaining their point of view to professionals, and professionals were getting the support to act. The Conference was followed by an *Update Report* two years later, checking out later the progress that had been made; that in turn was followed by another conference. Things were moving. And now, comes a new edition of Positive Smear.

There is still a long way to go. Rewriting huge swathes of

this book to bring it up to date, I am aware that women are still distressed and that professionals are still under-resourced to help them. New problems have arisen – the issue of instant treatment, and whether this puts even more emotional pressure on patients; renewed confusion for doctors (and hence for patients) around what the causes of cervical cancer really are. But at least now, the problems have been recognized, and we are tackling them.

So I want to say this. When I first wrote this book, I commented that I'd been accused of 'taking a risk . . . being too positive . . . expecting too much of women' in stating the hopeful side of having an abnormal smear, of asking women to learn from the experience. I still feel I was correct in my expectation – and more and more, over the years, I have been proved right. For increasingly, positive smear women I meet – at talks, conferences, at clinics or even at parties – are telling me that they have come through.

Sometimes they have hit rock bottom, in their panic or their anger; but they have been able to use the experience as a positive force in their lives. Women I have met have rethought their career direction; created new relationships; started families; begun getting healthy; become involved in pressure groups; recommitted themselves to having happy and fulfilled lives.

Faced with this evidence, then, even more than when *Positive Smear* was originally published, I believe the words I wrote then. 'We can take the good, even from something unpleasant. We can grow. We can make a difficult experience into a vital part of our lives and our development as human beings. We can turn a medical term on its head and truly make a 'positive smear' a 'positive experience'.

1   the process

1   Hearing the news

*' My doctor rang to say I had a
positive smear. It was as if a
friend had rung me up with the
news '*
(Linda)

You have had a smear test. Maybe because your Family Planning Clinic includes one in your check-up; maybe because you have had some bleeding and your doctor wants to make sure it is nothing serious; maybe because this is a regular part of your health care – for whatever reasons, you have had a smear test. You may or may not know exactly what it means, or what the results mean. You may or may not be aware of the implications, but you have had the test.

Unless your clinic is one that combines your smear test with further examination and can tell you immediately as you lie there what your result is, then you will have had to wait a while. (If your clinic is of this type, you may want to turn straight to Chapter 4, which deals with Diagnosis). Your wait may have been long – two weeks, four weeks, maybe two months. Perhaps you have put your smear test to the back of your mind, or perhaps it has been concerning you a bit.

Positive Smear

'I was pretending,' as one woman said, 'that I'd forgotten about it.' As the time goes by, you convince yourself that there is nothing wrong, and nothing to worry about.

Then comes the news. It might arrive in that 'little brown envelope', which when opened reveals a letter from your clinic or doctor. You might be one of the lucky women whose doctor phones them immediately the news comes through, or who gives them the news in person. You might not be so lucky. 'I got a message on my flatmate's telephone answering machine,' said Julia. Whichever way you hear the news, this is the beginning.

The news

What will the news say? Usually, it will be a straightforward statement that you have had a positive or 'abnormal' smear. It will remind you that you had a smear, and when, and also tell you to call into the doctor's surgery for a chat. Occasionally, your doctor or clinic will already have made a further appointment for you at a local hospital, and an appointment time and date will be given in the letter or phone call. Sometimes there may be a leaflet with the letter, explaining a little of the background to what has happened.

These are the bare bones of the news, but there are other messages locked into it too. Whoever is contacting you will want you to take your positive smear seriously, and might therefore use words like 'urgent' or 'at once'. Medical professionals, or their written material, may use medical terms, such as 'infection', 'pre-cancer' or 'dyskaryosis', terms you may not understand. It is also difficult sometimes, particularly during a phone call or consultation, to reconcile the businesslike message with what seems to be bad news. You may wonder what is really happening.

Some of the best messages contain a personal note from the doctor to you. Evelyn's doctor 'rang me immediately and said, "Look my dear, it's important that you go and have this seen to." I really appreciated that.' Doctors often do realize that women need to know what is happening and try to provide some understanding and reassurance right away. One woman's doctor wrote: 'Remember that smear tests are there to pick up changes *before* they get serious.' (Julie).

Some doctors are simply less sensitive, but you need to realize right from the start that at the other end of this news is a doctor who is human too. If s/he hasn't taken the time to word the message kindly or carefully, then that is his/her problem. It doesn't have to be yours.

First reactions

Many women report feeling shock as their first reaction: 'I just rushed into my flatmate's room and shrieked at him.' (Janet). You may actually feel the physical sensations of shock: shaking, clammy hands, breathlessness. Other women cope at first, and panic later: 'I kept thinking it was nothing to worry about; then I woke up in the middle of the night and thought – this must mean I'm dying.' (Diana). So if you are worried, if you have heard that a positive smear can mean treatment or serious illness and are panicked by this, then you are not alone. Many other women feel the same way.

At this stage, you may be unsure of how to react. You may

not know what having a positive smear is all about: 'It's so totally unknowable. You can't conceive of what it could actually mean.' (Rosemary). However you may be able to take the news calmly. If so, and if you can mobilize yourself into effective practical action, then this is the best possible way to be. Being calm, cool and powerfully active is going to get you furthest, fastest.

Other people

Other people around you when you receive the news will have to cope with you. If you do turn to them for support, remember two things. Firstly, if they don't know you well enough, they will find it difficult to give you exactly what you want. If a message reaches you at work, for example, other people might not know how to handle it. Illness, particularly sexual illness, stirs up strange things in people. It can also be appropriate to delay your reaction. I got my letter an hour before friends were coming round. After the first solitary weep, I decided not to tell my partner until after our friends had gone, when I could get the support I wanted for as long as I wanted. But also remember that other people are often only too glad to help. And other people may well learn from you that they too can ask for support when they need it.

What to do?

You have had the news, the first reactions are over, and you now need to begin to assimilate what is happening, and decide what to do next.

This is not something to be done with acquaintances or casual workmates. For this you need a friend, your partner, your Mum. If none of these are available, and you need to talk, you can contact a counselling network that will give you support over the phone; the Resource section in this book has plenty of ideas.

What are the issues you need to think through? The basic fact is that you have had a positive smear. This can mean a number of things. It could mean that you have a minor infection of the vagina or of the cervix which can be treated easily. It is also possible that you have an early pre-cancerous condition of the cervix which may need simple treatment or no treatment at all. There is a very slight possibility that you might have cancer, and if so there is an even slighter possibility that this might mean radical surgery.

It is easy at this stage for you, or other people, to suspect that you do have cancer and that you are going to die. There can also be a temptation to convince yourself that the doctors have made a mistake and that you can ignore the whole thing. Both of these possibilities are very unlikely. The truth is that the average family doctor will see only one case of invasive cancer and only two cases of advanced pre-cancer in their surgery every ten years – and you are unlikely to be one of these three people. The truth is that you probably don't have cancer. The truth is that you may not even need treatment. But it is also true that very few positive smear results are incorrect, and so you need to respond.

Of course, you don't *have* to go to the doctor or the hospital. It is possible to rip up the letter, ignore the phone call and

15

pretend it never happened. Quite a few of the women I talked to considered doing just that – although nowadays nationwide recall will mean that the system will, as one doctor so beautifully put it 'try to tempt you to come forward', by a letter, telephone call or visit.

But remember this. Someone, somewhere, has noticed that you are not as healthy as you could be. They have told you. They have given you the chance to do something about it. If they hadn't, your condition could be getting progressively worse and you would have no choice in the matter.

So maybe what you at first thought of as bad news is in fact good news.

2

What next?

*‘ My consultant looked at me
and said, ‘I think you may have
a problem . . .’ ’*
(Viki)

After you hear the news of your positive smear the next step
can vary enormously. Your doctor may have arranged an
examination for you at the local hospital. If so, turn to Chapter
3 where I describe this procedure. It is more likely that your
doctor will see you first, in order to talk about your smear
result.

The letter from your GP, Family Planning Centre or
Special Clinic will probably have included an appointment
date and time. If not, you have a choice: to go and see your
doctor, or to ring and ask to speak to her/him on the phone to
discuss your case. It is likely that the doctor will prefer to see
you in person, so don’t be disappointed or worried if the
receptionist asks you to make an appointment. It doesn’t mean
that the news is bad – your doctor simply thinks that seeing you
in person will be more helpful.

17

Positive Smear

Getting the results

Whether you see your doctor or speak on the phone, s/he is ideally placed to give you information about your case. By this time, particularly if you have been reading this book, you will probably have a good basic knowledge of what a positive smear means. If not, then ask your doctor to explain this to you.

If you haven't yet looked at the section of this book that deals with the facts about cervical conditions, I suggest you do so now, since you may find it useful for understanding what follows.

Smear result

The doctor will probably begin by telling you what your smear result is. The result will have been passed on to your doctor by means of a standard form, giving details of any abnormal changes in the cells and any other information picked up during the smear test. Remember that the doctor won't be able to tell you at this stage whether you have a serious condition, or give you any details about the condition you have; the smear test doesn't reveal this. However, depending on what degree of abnormal cell changes you have, the doctor will be able to advise you whether to have a further examination. Very often, with only a mild condition, you won't be referred for an examination at all; instead, the doctor will ask you to come back in three or six months for a repeat smear. If it seems likely that it is more than a mild condition, or if you have other symptoms or a history of cervical problems, the doctor will usually arrange a hospital appointment for you. S/he may do that there and then over the phone.

You need to be aware even at this stage whether, when you have your examination, there will be a possibility of immediate treatment in the hospital clinic. At present, only a few places in Britain offer this 'See and Treat' method, but if yours does, then your doctor will almost certainly know and be able to tell you. It is a good idea to check this, so that as you prepare for your examination, you also have a chance to prepare for the possibility of treatment.

The doctor will probably give you a letter to post or take to the hospital. 'Doesn't everyone steam the envelope open?' asked one woman – and you will have to decide whether you want to or not! Remember that it is your right to know what the doctors think your condition is, but also that there are better ways of finding out than being faced with a technical letter you can misunderstand. If you do want straight answers, try asking your doctor or consultant – at least that way you will have the chance to ask questions and have them answered, obtain information, and possibly even some support.

Often, this is all that a doctor does at this stage: gives you any information you need, and refers you to a specialist. The visit to the doctor might be very short indeed. Very occasionally, particularly if you have complained of particular symptoms and this has been the reason for your smear test, s/he will give you an internal examination. You probably will have had one before, but if not there's a fuller description of what it entails on page 35.

Infections

Sometimes, other cervical tests will have been done at the same time as your smear test. If an infection or virus has been

19

found, your doctor may take this opportunity to tell you about it.

Possible infections are thrush, trichomoniasis or chlamydia; you will probably be given cream to insert into your vagina, or tablets to take. If you have a virus, you may have to go to a specal clinic to have it treated, and your doctor will give you details of this. If, in fact, your smear has been done as part of your attending a special clinic, the doctor will be able to prescribe treatment for infections and viruses right away. Chapters 5-9 of this book include sections on these conditions and how they are treated. If you do have an infection, it may have made the smear result unclear and your doctor will ask you to have a repeat smear when the infection has been treated successfully.

Asking questions

Your doctor will usually give you all the information I have mentioned. It is useful, however, to take with you a check-list of questions to ask in case the doctor misses something you want to know about. Women I spoke to asked this kind of question during their visit:

> *What is my smear test result?*
> *What severity of condition have I got?*
> *Is there any other evidence to indicate what my condition is?*
> *Is there any sign of infection? A virus?*
> *Do I need to see a consultant? When? Where?*
> *How will the appointment be made?*

*Is there any chance that I will be offered treatment
    immediately after the examination (See and Treat)?
Do I need to come back to you for a repeat smear?
When?
Should I make the appointment now?*

Getting support

Whether you see your doctor in person or speak on the phone,
you may feel concerned when you contact her/him. You may
want to talk about your situation and be reassured. You have to
face the fact that some doctors will be quite happy to give you
the information you need, but will feel uneasy if you ask for
counselling or support. In an ideal world, of course, GPs
would have the opportunity and the energy to spend time with
you and let you express your worries.

Some of them do: 'My doctor was wonderful; he knew I'd
been depressed recently, and told me he accepted that I'd be
worried and that this was a bad time for a positive smear to
have happened.' (Julie).

If your doctor is like this, then do confide any fears you have
in him/her; s/he knows your medical and personal history and
is in an ideal situation to help you. If not, then the
responsibility is with you again, and you will have to find any
emotional support you need elsewhere.

Afterwards

Repeat smear

After your visit to the doctor, you may not need to attend a hospital, but will have been asked to return for a repeat smear after a short interval: don't be tempted not to. It is just as important (probably more so) to go for this smear as to go for the first one. Just because you have had a test doesn't mean to say that you are now safe for another three years; if the original test results were unclear, you need to have another as soon as you can.

Even if your doctor or FPC have said they will contact you when your next smear is due, this is never enough. They may forget, their records may go missing, or lightning may strike! If it does, and you miss a repeat smear, they won't suffer. You will.

As you leave the surgery or clinic, jot down in your diary the date when your repeat smear is due and mark in a date a few days before to remind you to arrange the test. The best time to go for a smear is at the mid-point of your menstrual cycle – that is, about twelve to sixteen days after the first day of your period. When the repeat smear is done, make sure you find the result; leave a stamped addressed envelope or ask when the result is likely to be in and ring back then. In this situation, where one smear has shown the need for a regular check on your health, you have every reason to have another.

Waiting

After visiting the doctor, you will probably know that the next stage is your hospital appointment. Here is where you may begin to learn the true (double) meaning of the word 'patient'. Waiting lists for such appointments can vary – depending on what your condition is and what part of the country you are in – from a few days to several months. You might be lucky and get an appointment fairly soon; this doesn't necessarily mean that you have a serious illness. Remember that doctors make their decisions about when to see you by considering the severity of your smear and your past medical history. I was seen within three days owing to the fact that both my parents had died of cancer, and despite the fact that at the time it seemed I only had a mild condition. If you develop any unusual bleeding or badly-smelling discharge, you will probably be seen quickly.

On the other hand, you may know that you have months to wait before you are examined and diagnosed, and this is very hard indeed. You may wonder whether your condition is getting worse, particularly as you don't yet know for sure what is the matter with you. Everyone I spoke to mentioned how difficult it was simply to wait: 'You never know what will happen . . . and you imagine the worst.' But remember that a large number of women who are referred for examination after one mildly abnormal smear (CIN1) will need no treatment at all – and that it is highly unlikely if you do need treatment that your condition will deteriorate badly while you wait. On the contrary, a recent study showed that some women's conditions showed a significant improvement between their smear test and further examination – though this does not mean, of course, that your examination is unnecessary. You, and your doctors, need it in order to know what is happening – and in order to decide what to do next.

Remember too, that waiting need not be a passive occupation. There are many things you can do to help yourself while you wait. One thing to do is to check that your appointment has been made. One woman I spoke to waited three months for her appointment, only to find that her GP's letter had been mislaid; her phone call alerted the hospital staff and she got an appointment soon after. There is no need to haunt the hospital, but it's worth asking your GP what the normal waiting time is and when he expects you to get an appointment. You can then ring the hospital when that time period has elapsed.

The other thing to do is to muster your forces. Get well-informed – read this book and any others in the Resource section that interest you. Spend time with people who can support you, as suggested in other chapters of this book. Build up your general health and well-being; whatever is the matter with you, you'll cope with the result far better if you are healthy and relaxed: 'I set up my own support system by doing intense relaxation, swimming, walking slowly . . . to strengthen my heart and relax me.' (Julie).

Finally, while you wait, keep your eyes and ears out for other women in the same situation. You'll be amazed at how many there are. One woman likened it to being pregnant: 'you find everyone else is too!' If you contact these other women, you can talk to them, support them and be supported by them.

As with pregnancy, the waiting is often the hardest part.

3   *The examination*

‘ *I got the works – the questions,*
the menstrual history, even a
breast examination. It was great! ’
(Julie)

In the positive smear process, hospital appointments are a bit like milestones; you seem to spend all your time waiting for, thinking about and heading for the next one. After the positive smear news itself, the next milestone will probably be a further examination. During the examination, the doctor will look at the evidence of your positive smear, and then do some further tests to find out what, if anything, is wrong.

Further examination can be carried out in a number of ways and which process you go through will depend very much on the area you live in and the resources that are available there. In addition, some methods of examination also include – or are used as methods of – treatment. In particular, recently, some hospitals may offer you See and Treat, diagnosing and treating you immediately after your examination.

The steps described below, as with all medical

25

examinations and treatments, may not be carried out in quite this order. Hospitals differ one from another in the way they go about examining – each has its own routine. So be prepared for your experience to be unique. The order in which this book describes events is only a basic framework into which you can fit your own chronology – of examination, diagnosis and treatment. Preparation, coping with waiting rooms, what happens in an internal examination – all these are constant throughout the process. Remember what is said about them here for reference later on. After your wait, this next step seems like the light at the end of a long tunnel, though you might feel scared and apprehensive about it.

There are two things you could feel apprehensive about: what the examination will be like, and its results. You may even find that all your negative feelings are being loaded on to one

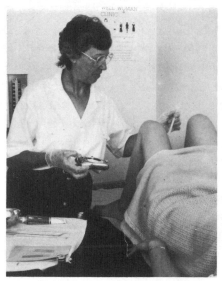

Figure 1 **Nurse taking a smear test**

26

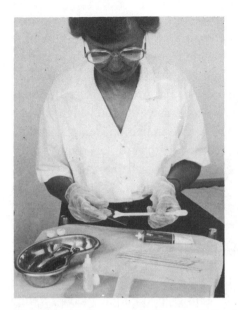

Figure 2 **Nurse preparing a slide from a smear test**

of these things, so that if asked, you will claim to be scared stiff about the examination – but in fact it is the results that really worry you.

Types of examination

These are the main types of examination used to investigate further. You may have just one before treatment, or you may need more than one – particularly if the abnormal cells have spread far up the cervical canal. Some health authorities don't have the facilities to do certain types of examination, so you may not have a choice.

Smear test: occasionally, further examination begins with a

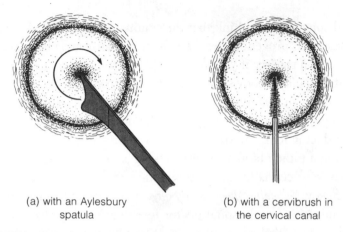

(a) with an Aylesbury
spatula

(b) with a cervibrush in
the cervical canal

Figure 3 **Taking a smear from the cervix**

smear test. This involves taking cells from your cervix and spreading them on a slide which will then be analysed to show any problems. It is a traditional method, developed in the 1940s by an Italian physician called Papanicolou, and the test is sometimes called a Pap smear, after him. Be clear, by the way, that the smear test does not in itself spot cancer; it only spots early cervical problems that may indicate cancer. A colposcopy and biopsy are needed in order for doctors to find out what is really happening.

Cervicography: this very new method of examination involves taking a photograph of your cervix which allows the doctor to take a very detailed look at the resulting slide under a microscope. Not many clinics offer this service yet, and it is used as an extension of the original smear test, to check if you need a follow-up by colposcopy and biopsy. It can have quite a high 'false positive' rate, meaning that you may be called back for further examination when in fact there is nothing wrong, and some doctors think that the trauma of being called back makes the procedure less worthwhile than a normal smear test. Don't worry if you are not offered this service; a smear test plus colposcopy serve the same purpose.

Colposcopy and punch biopsy: these are normally done at the same appointment, usually in Outpatients. In a colposcopy, the doctor looks at your cervix through a microscope on a stand; a punch biopsy involves taking a small sample of cells from your cervix for later examination.

Biopsy following loop diothermy: if, following an initial examination, the hospital doctor feels that s/he can go on to treat you with loop diothermy, (See Chapter 8) very often there will be no need to do an extra biopsy. The treatment itself allows the removed cells to be examined later, as would happen after any biopsy; the difference is that, with loop diothermy, you have already been treated, and the biopsy is simply used to check that no more serious problems exist. For more details on loop diathermy, turn to the chapter in this book on Treatment.

VABRA is a way of taking cells from the lining of your womb. It is usually an outpatient treatment, and is particularly useful for further investigation when you have heavy bleeding. It can also be done as an Inpatient examination when it is called a dilation and curretage (D and C).

Cane biopsy: a cone of tissue is taken from the cervix and this is often enough in itself to remove the abnormal cells as well as to diagnose them. However, if the biopsy shows invasive cancer, you will need further treatment. Cone biopsy usually involves a general anaesthetic and is used to investigate conditions where abnormal cells have spread, but

29

it can also be used as a form of treatment; because of this, I have chosen to deal with it in more detail later in this book in the chapter on treatment.

Which is the best sort of examination? In fact, they are all useful, depending on what your smear has shown, and what the doctor needs in order to find out what is the matter.

Preparations – at home

There are lots of ways that you can prepare for the examination. You may want to plan what to wear; a skirt is most sensible, since you can just slip off your underclothes when you are examined. Do check that your appointment doesn't clash with your period, for, as one woman I interviewed found to her cost, hospitals won't carry out some internal examinations if you are bleeding: ' I turned up, waited two hours, and then didn't even see a doctor when they heard I was having my period.' Equally, beware of douching or using a spermicide during intercourse just before your examination. This may confuse things, particularly any repeat smear that is taken.

You might like to have your partner or a friend with you at the hospital. Some things to consider when deciding who to take with you are the following: who will help me to feel as good as I can before and after the examination? Who will allow me to be myself, and express my feelings if I want to? Who can stand up to the doctors and ask the questions I want asked, if I'm feeling groggy or intimidated?

Once you have found someone to go with you (and made sure they can go on the day of your appointment), you might like to spend some time with them, talking about how you feel and how you might want them to support you. Also spend some time making out a list of questions you want to ask the doctor. Throughout this chapter – and indeed throughout the book – I will be suggesting questions for you to ask, and you can add specific ones of your own.

Preparations – at the hospital

It is likely that your examination will be at a local hospital, in the Outpatients Gynaecological Clinic. It is possible, though unlikely unless you live in a major city, that your GP, Family Planning Clinic or Special Clinic will be able to do the examination themselves.

When you arrive at the hospital and find your way to the clinic mentioned on your appointment card, you will probably have to check in at the reception desk after which you will probably have to wait. Many women I talked to complained about the waiting times for all kinds of diagnosis and treatment. This is certainly not something unique to gynaecological clinics – but waiting is always soul-destroying when you are waiting to hear what is wrong.

'All these women sitting round, too frightened to talk to one another', was how one interviewee described it. Perhaps there is a better way, if we realize that every woman there is probably in the same position as ourselves – or further down the treatment line. Talking to them can help you feel better, and make all of us feel less alone. A waiting-room full of women supporting each other by exchanging information, reassurance and help is a power-house of useful energy; tap into it if it exists, and if not, be the one to start it.

31

To undress or not

Once you are called by the nurse, you will have to negotiate the problem of undressing. Exactly what this involves will vary from hospital to hospital and from doctor to doctor. Many doctors nowadays insist on seeing all their patients fully dressed to begin with: as one doctor put it, this 'creates an atmosphere of respect'. Not all hospitals are so enlightened, however: there are many horror stories of women clad in short white ward gowns 'with the back flapping open to show my bottom', having to wait on wooden seats for hours, embarrassed and chilly.

If you find yourself in this situation, you have two choices. You can refuse point blank to undress completely, and insist on being examined with just your briefs and tights off. If anyone argues, call in your friend or partner as support and simply stay calm and friendly – without removing your clothes. Or you can tell the nurse that you are very happy to undress, but will only do it just before the doctor is ready to see you. Ask her/him to let you know which patient is seeing the doctor before you, and then wait fully dressed until that patient goes in. Then get changed. The hour spent fully dressed and therefore feeling less vulnerable will be well worth it.

A final tip – whether you go in to see the doctor dressed or undressed, make sure you have your briefs with you, since you may need them later in order to wear a sanitary towel.

Meeting the consultant

Don't be overawed by any medical professional. Ask for your

friend or partner to be there if you want them to be, and remember that it is worth your while to create an equal relationship right from the start. You can begin to do this by asking some questions right away. Some questions that women I talked to asked at this point were these:

> *What is your name? What sort of doctor are you? What*
>   *job do you do in the hospital?*
> *What is the nurse's name? Will she stay in the room with*
>   *me?*
> *What has my GP/clinic said to you in the letter?*
> *Are you going to take another smear? Photograph of my*
>   *cervix? Colposcopy? Biopsy?*
> *Will I have the opportunity for treatment now if your*
>   *examination suggests that is possible?*
> *Will there be anyone else in the room while I'm being*
>   *examined?*

The last question can be more relevant than it seems: Julie's doctor began to examine her while students were in the room. She objected to this, and requested that they leave, which they did. You may feel, like Julie, that your medical condition and your body are something you only want to share with the doctor and nurse. On the other hand, you may like to let students learn from your situation; students do require training if we are to have the doctors of tomorrow. Whatever the case, a consultant should check with you before allowing students into the room, and you do have every right to refuse if you want to.

Doctor's questions

At this stage, the doctor will probably have some questions to ask

33

you. They will often be about your gynaecological history to help the doctor understand what is going on in your cervix, and to have a context in which to interpret what s/he is seeing when s/he examines you. It is therefore worth answering them as fully as possible. You could perhaps prepare for them beforehand by making sure you know such things as: the date of your last period; the dates of your pregnancies; whether you are pregnant at the moment; whether there is any history of cancer in your family.

Some questions might embarrass you, however, and you may not want to answer them: the age at which you first had intercourse, or the number of sexual partners you have had are personal issues and you may think of them as things you want to keep to yourself. In addition, of course, many of these questions presuppose not only that your sexual relationship includes penetration, but also that it is with a male partner. Even if you have found the courage to be totally open about your sex life with friends and family, it may be difficult to explain to a total stranger that you are celibate or lesbian; if you have not yet confided in anyone about your situation, such questions may be distressing to you. Forewarned is forearmed, however; remember that all judgments about your sex life are solely a result of social prejudice – they are other people's problem, not yours. And remember that you don't have to answer if you don't want to.

Equally, even if you find the questions you are asked unobjectionable, it is worth asking whether the doctor needs to know the answers to such questions in order to diagnose your condition. While it is very likely that s/he does, it is also possible that the questions are part of a larger issue – perhaps gathering information for a survey. Such surveys are of great

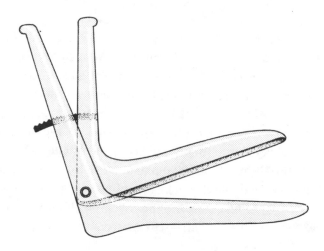

Figure 4 **A speculum is a plastic or metal instrument which looks like two shoe horns joined together**

use in detecting trends in cervical conditions and cancer, and it is important that women take part in them, but of course they are not related to your cure. So if a question causes you particular embarrassment, it is worth checking whether you really do need to reply to it.

The internal examination

The doctor will usually have read your notes and looked at the results of your positive smear. Then s/he will give you an internal examination. You will most likely have had one before, when you had your smear, but here is a detailed description. If you need further treatment, then you will have many more internals to come.

First you need to get into a position where the doctor can

see inside your cervix. This usually means lying flat on your back on an examining couch with your legs raised and parted. There are special stirrups for your legs to rest on, which can be 'twigs on sticks' as one woman described them, or canvas or plastic slings into which your legs fit. This position can be off-putting; it may also make you feel vulnerable. But one woman's realization could help: 'Remembering that I was in charge helped a lot. I kept telling myself that I had chosen to be there because I wanted to be healthy – and that that meant I was in control.' (Tracey).

If you feel uncomfortable, do say so, and get the leg-rests adjusted. Feeling embarrassed does not mean you are what

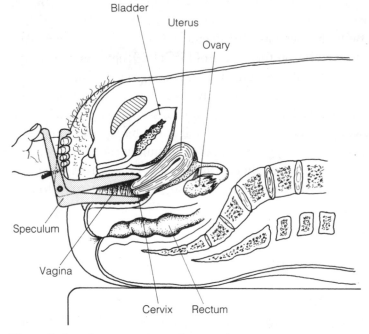

Figure 5 **As the speculum is eased apart, it opens your vagina so that the doctor can see inside it**

one interviewee called 'a nuisance patient'; lots of women feel this way, though do remember that although you are an individual to the doctor, you are not a sexual object.

When you are settled, the doctor will place a metal or plastic instrument called a speculum into your vagina. You will almost certainly have had one used in your smear test. The speculum looks rather like two shoe horns joined together and as it is eased apart, it opens your vagina so that the doctor can see down to your cervix.

As with all these examinations and treatments, there is no promise that this will not be uncomfortable; however, it is usually just cold. If you are uncomfortable, you might try asking your friend, or the nurse, to hold your hand or talk to you to distract you. One doctor in London has music playing and pictures on the ceiling of his colposcopy clinic – perhaps you should start a campaign for similar facilities in your area.

The full examination may take as long as ten or fifteen minutes, so don't panic if the doctor seems to be taking a close look. The doctor will often tell you what s/he's doing as it happens. If not, you can ask for a running commentary if you want one, though there will probably be a period when the doctor needs to concentrate and so may not want to talk to you.

The examination

Smear test

With your vagina open, the doctor will probably begin by taking another smear to see if the result is still the same. There have been cases of cervical conditions clearing up between one smear and the next. S/he will scrape a spatula or brush around your cervix in a complete circle, trying to make sure that s/he has gathered a sample of all the cells around the neck of the womb. The doctor or nurse will then spread the cells on to a glass slide, which is stained so that individual cells can be easily seen. This is then examined under a microscope (when you have your smear taken by your GP or clinic nurse, this examination is done later in a special testing laboratory by a specially trained technician). The smear, as I have pointed out, may highlight a number of possibilities, including inflammation, infections, viruses and abnormal cells. It cannot, however, tell you whether severely changing cells are yet invasive.

Cervicography

This procedure, in which a photograph is taken of your cervix,

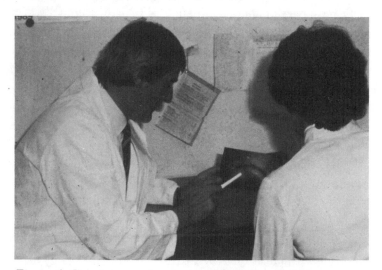

Figure 6 **Cervicography: examining the picture**

is very similar to a smear test. Your vagina is opened by a speculum as usual and then a mild and painless solution of acetic acid is applied to your cervix. The process of placing a camera at the entrance to your vagina takes only a few minutes, and the camera should not even touch you while the photograph is being taken, after which the film is sent away for development. When it returns, the doctor will check the slide under magnification for evidence of abnormal cells. 'The waiting is the worst; what will they find?' commented Jan. The method does have the advantages of being easy, quick and totally painless – though as mentioned before, it can tend to show false positives.

Colposcopy

The next part of the examination is usually colposcopy. In colposcopy, the doctor looks at your cervix through a microscope on a stand. S/he examines the surface appearance of your cervix very closely, to see whether there are any signs of abnormality, and if there is any evidence of other problems. Remember that the doctor cannot tell from colposcopy how far or how deep the disease has spread, or whether it is cancerous.

First, s/he will put a liquid on your cervix: this may be a solution of acetic acid or iodine, so it could sting a bit. The abnormal areas turn a different colour, making them easier to see.

The doctor will then place the colposcope (microscope) at the entrance to your vagina, and will look closely at your cervix. In some clinics it is now possible for you to see what the doctor sees on closed circuit television. If you are able to see your cervix on camera, it will look strange. Your vagina may look huge, and the coloured problem areas may also look very large. You need to put this into perspective: what you are seeing is only a very small proportion of your cervix, and the healthy areas of cells will far outweigh any non-healthy areas. Similarly, problem areas may not be abnormal cells, but only simply-treated infections, though they may well look the same to you on camera.

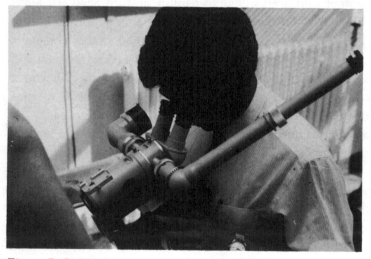

Figure 7 **Colposcopy**

Punch biopsy

The next stage is usually for the doctor to take a small sample of the cervical cells for the laboratory to examine under a microscope. This is a normal thing to do, and does not mean you have cancer, so don't panic if the doctor talks about taking a 'biopsy'.

The doctor takes a tiny snippet of cells from your cervix, and will sometimes take more than one sample. It is hard to predict whether you will feel any pain at this stage, since it depends on a number of things: your doctor's sensitivity, your reaction to pain, the size and number of the samples doctors like to take. One woman described it as being 'like a bad period pain', another said 'it wasn't at all painful, and I'd been warned it would be.' One very positive suggestion reported in *The Lancet*[1] was that if warned at the exact moment that a biopsy is taken, you can cough, which tenses you against the pain and also distracts you. Try asking your doctor to give you a count-down to the 'snip', and also to tap the inside of your thigh as s/he cuts; this will hopefully both reduce any discomfort and give you a feeling of involvement in what is happening.

You might bleed however, and the nurse will probably give you a sanitary towel to put on afterwards. This is the reason for the earlier warning about making sure you have your briefs with you. Few things are more awkward than sitting clutching said towel while talking to the doctor, and at the same time 'feeling sticky underneath', as one woman put it.

When the biopsy is over, the doctor will usually go to wash her/his hands, while the nurse helps you out of the stirrups and down from the couch. If you haven't had your friend with you up to now, this is the time to ask him or her to come in while you talk to the doctor after the examination.

As mentioned earlier, the kind of in-depth examination of cervical cells that a punch biopsy makes possible is also part of having loop diothermy treatment. The process itself is as described in Chapter 8 – and has the advantage over many other treatments that the cells which are removed from your cervix remain intact, and can be taken away to be examined. If there seem to be any problems that have not already been treated, this biopsy will make them clear, and you can then be brought back for further treatment.

What now?

Once the examination is over, the doctor may have enough information to be able to tell you what is wrong. If examination has been combined with treatment, s/he may even be able to tell you that you are cured and need only come back for a check-up – always providing your biopsy has shown up nothing more serious. But often, your doctor may not be able to give you a definite diagnosis immediately after the examination. S/he may want to wait for the results of a biopsy. S/he may want to consult with another doctor. S/he may even want you to come back for further examination because s/he has not yet got all the information s/he needs. If you don't get a diagnosis at once, it certainly doesn't mean that something is seriously wrong. However, because examination and diagnosis are often two separate things, I have separated them into two chapters in this book.

Afterwards

Physical reactions

After the examination, your physical reactions might range

from feeling nothing at all to feeling quite sore, especially after a biopsy. It is not a good idea to try to travel by bicycle, for obvious reasons, and it is probably wise to give yourself some time in case you need to sit down and collect yourself before you attempt the journey back home or to work.

On the other hand, you may be one of the lucky women who simply bounces back and feels no after-effects. This is quite normal; the important thing to remember is that if you do feel physically vulnerable after the examination, this is quite normal, too. If for any reason, after such an examination, you start bleeding heavily when you are not due to have your period, then see your GP or ring the hospital for advice.

In particular, if you are, or suspect you may be pregnant, go immediately to your doctor if you find any nasty after-effects from examination. It is very rare for any of the processes I mention to cause problems, but one can never by too careful. A few women reported that after the examination, their consultant advised them not to make love for a while. Doctors usually use this term to mean not having penetrative sex – and you may want to bear in mind that enjoyable love-making need not, of course, involve penetration at all!

Emotional reactions

Women's feelings about the examination also varied enormously: 'It didn't hurt, but it was bloody embarrassing,' said one woman. 'When you've had three children, it's not such an invasion of your privacy,' said another.

If you dislike having an internal examination, you may feel intruded upon. If it was painful, you might feel tearful and angry. You may have objected to having a doctor (particularly a male doctor) examining intimate parts of your body. You may have been wary of how the doctor will respond to your genitals; female circumcision, for example, can trigger quite distressed or critical reactions in doctors who are unused to it. It may be that an internal examination creates negative feelings in you because it is so like penetrative sex; whether you are heterosexual or lesbian, you may have chosen not to include penetration in your current sexual relationship, or the memory of earlier penetrative sex may be upsetting for you.

If your examination does trigger strong feelings for you, then next time you go for an examination, or when you go for later treatment, make sure you have special support – a friend to fight for your rights, your lover to hold your hand. Make sure too that you have a chance both before and after your hospital visit to express the hurt you feel, not only about what is happening here and now, but about past memories that have created your emotional vulnerability. Such support can give you the opportunity to explore the feelings you have, and maybe resolve them to some extent, for next time you have a gynaecological problem. The important thing to remember here is that simply because the doctor is trying to help you, it doesn't mean that you have to feel totally positive about everything; your feelings are yours and you need to respect them.

You might, though, be one of the women I talked to who in fact found something good in the experience. It helps if you can go into the whole experience determined to find such things: were you surprised at how supportive your friend was; satisfied with the doctor's explanations; did you get on with the other women in the waiting room?

Above all, did the doctor learn anything? Can s/he now, armed with the information s/he has gained, go on to diagnose if anything is wrong – and so begin to help you towards health?

4

The diagnosis

*' When they told me the
diagnosis, I burst into tears. The
doctor said 'Well, you must have
known something was wrong.' '*
(Sue)

T he first thing to say about the diagnosis is that it won't
necessarily take place at the same time as the examination.
Often it does. The colposcopy over, the doctor can sit down
with you and explain just what is happening, suggest treatment
and send you away with all questions resolved. But it doesn't
always happen like this.

The doctor may ask you to come back in a few weeks' time.
As always, the waiting list can vary, and I found examples of
women delayed anything up to seven weeks for examination
results. It is usual for women in this situation to be asked to
come back to the same clinic, where they can see a consultant
(though be warned, it might not be the same consultant);
unlike smear or pregnancy results, you won't usually be told
over the phone.

Whether you get your diagnosis immediately or after a

while, make sure you are well prepared. You may want to read the chapter in this book on Facts, in order to have a background to what the doctor is saying to you, and particularly in order to understand any technical words s/he is using. You may want to take a friend or partner with you, for support. When you first enter the consulting room, as I suggested in the chapter on examination, spend a few minutes making contact with the doctor. Then you are ready to go on to discuss the diagnosis.

Diagnosis

Working together

Remember that the doctor's diagnosis is only an external comment on your health. It can be tempting to place all the responsibility on the doctor, to wait to be told what is the matter with you; but you don't have to hand over total control like this.

In fact, you will probably have thought about what might be the matter with you. Many women 'knew there was something wrong' – tiredness, feeling out of sorts, an awareness of 'lack of balance' as one woman described it, could have indicated that you were not well.

So maybe we can move towards a situation where patient and doctor can work together to arrive at a diagnosis. In many ways, we already do; the doctor asks you questions about your medical history, and you tell her/him about your symptoms. We all go to the diagnosis with some idea, right or wrong, of what we think is the matter.

Try taking things a stage further than this. Before you see your doctor, spend some time considering your body, becoming aware of any symptoms you have, and what feelings you have noticed. It could be that nothing comes to mind or else you might gradually become conscious of what is wrong with you. If you have had definite symptoms, such as vaginal discharge or bleeding, then try to remember when, how much and of what type; for example, do you bleed after intercourse? (many women do so without having cancer); is your vaginal discharge clear or coloured? Remember that you might have a tendency to think the worst about what is happening to you, and so try to be aware of when you are offering useful information – 'I've noticed that I have pain on intercourse, but only at certain times of the month' – and when you are simply panicking.

Then, when you are with the consultant, try asking whether the doctor would be interested in hearing your opinions about your condition. If your doctor is willing, tell her/him what feelings you have noticed, any symptoms you have identified, what your instincts tell you. If the doctor listens, s/he will learn a great deal, and may be able to make a more accurate diagnosis. You will have taken a part in what is happening, rather than simply waiting to be told what is the matter with you.

Questions and answers

At this point, the doctor will begin to discuss your diagnosis, hopefully in language you can understand. Do ask for explanations of terms that you are not familiar with. Maybe s/he will show you a photograph of your cervix, showing the normal and abnormal cells, or draw a diagram to demonstrate where the abnormality is and how far it has spread. This is the time to ask further questions. Remember that if you have just had your examination and are feeling a bit shaky, your friend can ask the questions for you. Some questions women asked were these:

> *What exactly did you find during your examination?*
> *What was my repeat smear/cervicography result?*
> *What did the biopsy show?*
> *What grade of CIN do I have?*
> *How far has it spread?*
> *Can you tell me now whether my condition is*
> *cancerous or precancerous?*

Remember to ask the doctor to explain again anything you don't understand. There may be pressure on her/him to complete your appointment quickly, because there are other people waiting, but for you this is an important opportunity to confer with a professional who knows your condition – so take it.

You may not only want to know about your CIN condition. It might be important for you and for your partner to know about any other conditions of your cervix. Even if no treatment is needed, there might be some sort of infection or virus that you should know about so that you can deal with it.

So further questions to ask are:

> *Did you notice any inflammation of my cervix? Do*
> *you know what might be causing this?*
> *Was there any vaginal discharge? Can you suggest*
> *what might be causing this?*
> *Did you find any evidence of infection or viruses?*

50

Possibilities

All clear

It is possible that after a preliminary positive smear result, a few weeks or months later you show no signs of abnormal cells. This is possibly the best news of all. It shows what is now being accepted by medical professionals: that although all cervical conditions need attention, many, particularly at the level of CIN1, will get better by themselves.

However, you do need to look at what in your life made you vulnerable to developing the abnormal cells in the first place. If you do this – perhaps by reading the chapters in this book on causes and on prevention – you may find that in order to make yourself less vulnerable in the future, you need to change something about your life.

Cervical problems

You may well have cervical problems other than those that a smear test is specifically designed to spot. If so, your consultant may want to discuss them with you. You will probably have been told by your GP about any infections or viruses you may possibly have. The consultant may add an extra comment about them, or suggest you have them treated if you aren't doing so already. If s/he does not, you should mention them; any cervical condition needs to be resolved as soon as possible if you are to have full cervical health – and it is a good idea to insist, even if your doctor doesn't, that this is done before treatment for your abnormal smear. You may also want to explore, if you haven't already done so, getting treatment for any infection or virus you have that may affect your partner.

Equally, if the consultant notices that you have a cervical ectropion (erosion), s/he may tell you this. Remember that, as explained in the chapter on Facts, this condition is not serious, and may not need treatment at all.

CIN (cervical intraepithelial neoplasia) or abnormal cell change

It is almost certain that your positive smear is due to a pre-cancerous condition of the cervix. So the likelihood is that the doctor will tell you that you have a CIN condition, grades 1, 2 or 3. This means, as we see in Chapter 8, that you have some cells on your cervix that are abnormal and treatable. You may not even need treatment, if the condition is in the early stages. More and more, nowadays, women are being offered the option of leaving CIN1 conditions untreated and having them monitored instead; they may go away. With CIN2 and 3, this is not a wise thing to do, and your doctor will not offer you this option.

If yours is a CIN1 condition, then the most logical thing for you to do is to jump up and down in the consulting room shouting for joy. For you are one of the majority of women in whom a pre-cancerous condition has been spotted in good time. And once you have treated the condition, you have a high chance of never being bothered with it again. That is the logic of the situation.

However, we are not logical beings. Straightforward as the medical facts are, we can still feel upset, frightened and angry. We have brains and emotions, and they get carried along too.

So if you are diagnosed like this, and you still feel a bit weepy or at a loss, or if you are still worried about treatment or other people's reactions, you are perfectly normal – and you are not alone.

'After my colposcopy I was told: "the cells are abnormal, but don't worry." I didn't worry. I was concerned.' (Judith).

'I was clear from the start that it was never cancer. I think I coped well, but I did get down sometimes, for other reasons.' (Evelyn).

What if it is cancer?

Your doctor may tell you that you have cervical cancer. The thing to remember is that it is highly unlikely that you will die. The annual death rate from cervical cancer is 2,000 (as compared to 15,000 women a year who die of breast cancer). However, remember that 85 per cent of women who have cervical cancer have never had a smear; of the 15 per cent left, most have only ever had one smear. The fact that you have, that your condition has been noticed through an examination, rather than left to become more advanced, means that you have more than a very good chance of total recovery. Mostly, nowadays, cancer does not kill.

I spoke in my interviews to three women who had had cervical cancer. They had all had hysterectomies, two had had radical radiotherapy. All three have now passed the five year 'all-clear' point, and I can testify that they are all energetic, powerful, vital women. These are some of the things they said to me:

'Since then, I've been on an assertiveness course for women. I've learned to ask for what I want.' (Sue).

'Yes, my life did change . . . I worry so much less now.' (Jane).

These women are not in any way saying that if you have cervical cancer then everything is fine. What they are saying is that it is not the end.

It is possible, at this point, that if you have had cancer diagnosed, you will need to supplement this book with other sources of information. You are travelling a different path from most of the women who have a positive smear. If you look in the Resource section of this book, you will find a full list of many of the support services for cancer, and a long list of books written especially for you and your problems and challenges.

Pregnancy

A few of the women I spoke to had been pregnant when they discovered that they had a cervical condition. A smear test is often routine in the first stages of pregnancy, and this can be the time that your cervical condition is first spotted.

This is a difficult situation and merits talking through carefully with your doctor. Remember first of all that it can be difficult to interpret the results of smear tests taken during pregnancy, because the particular hormones flooding your body may confuse the issue. It can be that with mild conditions, there is, in fact, no real problem at all, and that after your pregnancy is over, your cervix will return to normal. So your doctor may advise you to wait until your first period after pregnancy, perhaps three months or so, and have a repeat smear before coming to a certain diagnosis. But even if the signs are of a more advanced pre-cancer condition, it is also likely that you will be advised not to have treatment until after you have given birth. This may concern you. But remember that often there is no danger to yourself or your baby in leaving your condition untreated; if you went through the normal medical system, it is possible you would have to wait months for treatment anyway, so you are in no worse a position.

If your condition is more serious, then you will need to take some informed decisions. Developing cervical cancer when pregnant is rare, so I am not going to dwell on it in too much detail. However you may have to face up to the fact that a normal pregnancy and cervical cancer are not easily compatible, and that you have to choose between them.

On the other hand, two of the women I talked to who had cervical abnormality were advised to go through with their pregnancies and have a hysterectomy immediately afterwards. Your doctor will be able to talk through with you exactly what your decisions should be.

Match or mismatch?

Usually, your idea of what is wrong with you and the doctor's diagnosis agree. You respect her/his professional ability and you know in your heart that what s/he says is right, whether you like it or not. It can sometimes happen though that your diagnosis and the doctor's don't match. You feel your condition is not what s/he says it is. Look at these feelings carefully. You may have been so upset by the diagnosis that you are refusing to believe it. However if you calmly and coolly believe that you are right and the diagnosis is wrong, then this is an opportunity to look after yourself in the best way possible. There are several things you can do about a mismatch between your instincts and your doctor's diagnosis.

You might be tempted to ignore the diagnosis completely; this is never a good thing to do. 'I thought – if I just go home, and not let them touch me, then it will all go away.' (Sue). Fortunately, Sue didn't just go home, and she did survive cervical cancer.

You can challenge your doctor. You can ask her/him to examine you again and see if your condition is still the same. The condition might have retreated, and before you progress to treatment, you will want to be sure you really need it. Another option is to ask for a second opinion, or change doctors completely. Heather was dissatisfied with her doctor's diagnosis that her cervical condition was not serious and could be left untreated for six months. She went back to the clinic with a friend, and demanded another smear. Her condition had worsened; she then fought for, and received, laser treatment.

Diagnosis – right and responsibility

The vast majority of diagnoses are correct – and in the over-strained health service, we shouldn't let simple panic or distress push us to illogical demands on the medical profession. However if you do believe that your diagnosis is wrong, then to challenge it is your right – and your responsibility.

In the long term, after the positive smear diagnosis is in the past, you can learn from the whole experience to take notice of what your body is saying and begin to take responsibility for its health. You can become more conscious of when you are ill, and when you are truly well. You can begin to diagnose your own physical state, using the doctor to confirm or make more accurate what you have found out for yourself. Then you will have learned something, you will have increased your chances of health in the future. And in the interim you will be able to move on towards treatment and towards cure.

5   Which treatment – alternative ways

' All this aggressive treatment ...
isn't there a better way? '
(Tracey)

Your condition has been diagnosed. All that remains is for you to have the condition 'zapped away' as one consultant put it. In fact, I don't think that it need be like this. I think that there is a case for stopping and thinking. The consultant has her/his own pattern of recommending treatment. S/he does it all in good faith, and is usually correct. Your view is a little different. Yours is the only case you have to think about at the moment. You have little professional expertise, but when the treatment is over, you are the person who has to live with the consequences. So stopping and thinking is often a good idea.

For there is a pattern, even in the early stages of CIN, of recommending strong, 'aggressive' treatment as a matter of course – diathermy, cone biopsy, cryosurgery. There is a temptation to 'zap and discharge' a patient, and in many cases this is the only alternative for doctors who are concerned that if they offer gentler forms of treatment the condition will spread or the patient simply never return for check-ups. With your awareness, and your concern for yourself, maybe you have other alternatives.

A word of warning is needed here. The more advanced your condition, the further along the scale of CIN-cancer you are, the less time you have to stop and think, and the more advisable standard treatment is. I am not suggesting (for those panicking medical professionals who think I am) that you go home and allow yourself to die of advanced invasive cancer with secondaries.

But in Britain today, we have a situation in which the waiting list for diagnosis, not to mention the treatment, is often of several months. This scandal can actually be quite good news for those of us who prefer to try gentler methods of treatment before agreeing to more aggressive methods such as laser. I would suggest that we could use this time to do something ourselves.

Many of the women I spoke to did this. Jane G. had laser treatment but supported it with homoeopathy for 'the anxiety, the bruising and shock. When I went back, the surgeon commented on how well I'd healed.'

This chapter then, covers some alternative, less invasive approaches that you may choose to use yourself, particularly if you have CIN1 and 2, before agreeing to hospital treatment. Remember that in such cases it can be better to go for the total health of the body rather than for the total destruction of a few rogue cells.

Treatment choices

Do nothing

This is not really a viable option. The particular circumstances

60

that made you vulnerable to the cervical condition are probably still present, and unless something happens, the changing cells on your cervix will continue to change. So *never* ignore it. It won't go away.

Build health

You can try and prevent cervical conditions developing by being as healthy as you can be, and you can also support whatever treatment you receive in the same way. Building health won't suddenly create spontaneous remission of any disease you have – but it will allow you to get better more quickly, and it is something you can do all by yourself.

What should you be doing? Your aim is to become as healthy as you can in a fairly short time, without straining an already vulnerable system. There are several ways to build health, and many books on the subject and the chapter in this book on Prevention outlines some of the ways you can build health long-term.

Changes to diet can't be made overnight, but you can cut down on obviously harmful things, and increase your intake of obviously beneficial things. Many reports now link diets rich in fat, salt and alcohol with cell changes similar to the ones found in abnormal conditions of the cervix – so try reducing your intake of these three things. And even in the short time it may take for you to be booked in for treatment, it will do no harm to switch to non-refined foods, cut down on sugar, avoid tea and coffee. These changes will not bring about a cure by themselves, but they may make it easier for your body to heal itself.

61

It is also advisable, particularly if you are going to have a general anaesthetic, to work on improving your lung power. Don't suddenly leap into an intensive jogging programme when you haven't even run for a bus for the last two years. Take regular, gentle exercise; frenetic activity such as looking after two under-fives doesn't count, by the way! Try swimming as one woman did: 'to feel my body was participating in getting more healthy'. Relax for a few minutes several times a day. Do lots of things you enjoy and that make you feel good.

Vitamins and minerals

There are several dietary elements that are often absent in women with cervical cancer and CIN conditions. Recent work done in America has suggested that taking regular doses of these in early cases of cervical abnormality may prove useful, and a new study at the British Imperial Cancer Research Fund (see Resource section) is currently underway, where volunteers with CIN1 are asked to take a daily vitamin tablet containing Vitamins C, E and beta carotene.

Vitamin C seems to convert toxic substances in the blood into harmless ones which are then passed out of your body in your urine; the levels of the substance appear to be lower than usual in abnormal cervical cells. Try to eat more citrus fruits and uncooked vegetables, and supplement your diet with Vitamin C tablets; 100 mg is the recommended daily amount, though some doctors say that 10 g is standard cancer therapy. It is not a case of more is better, though; although there are no serious side-effects if you overdose, you may find yourself with diarrhoea.

Folic acid is found in yeast, wheatgerm, nuts and pulses. It can also be taken as a supplement, and one recommended dose is 10 mg a day. Oral contraceptives can create folic acid deficiency, so if you are on the Pill you might like to try taking a supplement, although again, too much is not a good idea.

Beta carotene, found particularly in carrots, green leafy vegetables, apricots and peaches, is another possible treatment. One woman started drinking carrot juice from the time of her smear up to the time of her laser treatment – and claims it improved her eyesight too. There is a danger of overdosing however, so as a general rule two glasses a day will do. Large doses of synthetic beta carotene or vitamin A need to be taken under supervision, though the amounts included in most multivitamin pills are safe – as long as you stick to the recommended dosage.

Give up smoking

Whilst giving up smoking has obvious long-term benefits, and so is a natural step if you wish to prevent cervical problems (see Chapter 7), recent research suggests that particularly for early conditions, it can be a treatment too. A current study at the Imperial Cancer Research Fund, for example, asks women with CIN1 to give up smoking and see if that has an effect on their condition (see Resource section). So you may want to try giving up smoking and see if, by the time you come to have treatment, your condition has improved or even reversed itself.

Barrier contraception

The chapter on Causes explains how using barrier contraception may decrease vulnerability in your cervix. Using a barrier method is not only a good way to prevent, but also to treat your condition. In an American study of 135 women with abnormal cervical cells, 133 of them got better spontaneously simply by their partner using a condom over a period of several months[2]. This amazingly simple and trouble-free way of curing cervical problems seems to have been largely ignored by medical professionals in the West and I do wonder why; perhaps they are frightened it won't work, or perhaps it just seems too easy. It also places the control back in the patient's hands, which is sometimes hard for doctors to handle.

Naturally, I am not suggesting that using barrier contraception will cure all CIN conditions. Nor would I suggest that using a condom and never going back for a repeat smear is the answer. Changing to barrier methods might anyway be difficult for you and your partner, for a number of reasons, but do look carefully at the advantages.

If you have a positive smear, try using a barrier method of contraception immediately. If you have been told simply to come back for a repeat smear, use it until then. If you have a more severe condition on the CIN grade, then in the intervals between the news and the diagnosis and treatment, try using a barrier method. During further examination, a repeat smear may well reveal that your condition has now cleared up.

If your condition proves to need further treatment, you have lost nothing at all by using barrier contraception. And you can choose to have that treatment just as before. If you have in fact cured yourself, then congratulations. You've avoided the upset to your body of further treatment. Tell your consultant and everyone else about your success in a loud voice. A further reason for using contraception (whether it be barrier contraception or another method) once you have had a positive smear, is that it is vitally important not to get pregnant while you are waiting for treatment. Your being pregnant may confuse any diagnosis, and treatment is difficult while you are pregnant.

Remember that after you have a clear result, you need to consider the issues involved before deciding whether to stop using barrier contraception.

Clearing up infections

Infections can mask other conditions of the cervix, so you should get them cleared up as soon as you can. You can ask your doctor for treatment for yourself, and your partner if necessary, if s/he hasn't already suggested this. There is a range of strong antibiotics to treat most vaginal infections, and they are often quick and effective. You may want to think carefully before taking antibiotics, however, because they do lower your immunity to infection and they can stay in your bloodstream for a long time afterwards. Depending on what your particular infection is, there are sometimes more natural alternatives available; the leaflets, books and contacts in the Resource section will give you further help with this.

Clearing up viruses

If you have any viruses, you will also want to get these treated too. Usually your doctor will have been alerted to their possibility on the first smear and offered you treatment. If not, the consultant may have mentioned them after your colposcopy. If you know you have any viruses and doctors do not mention treating them, then as I suggested before, make the first move towards treatment by mentioning this yourself. Remember that if you are to stay virus-free, both you and your partner need to be treated.

Most common viruses can clear up spontaneously, and if you are healthy and stress-free, then this is more likely to happen. However you may need to obtain medication or treatment from your doctor or to attend a special clinic. Don't be put off by the fact that the special clinic is for sexually transmitted diseases – this very fact means that the staff will probably be more at ease with your condition than your doctor is.

Herpes. Whilst current medical thought plays down the direct link between cervical pre-cancer and the herpes virus, your smear test may have drawn attention to the possibility of your having it. Things to do for yourself are: wash often and gently, avoiding soap; do not wear anything that can irritate the herpes such as tight briefs or nylon. Increase your zinc intake with a mineral supplement, taking care not to exceed the recommended amount. If the herpes is painful, take pain-killers. Current orthodox treatment offered by hospitals includes drugs that seem to relieve the symptoms and reduce the chances of another attack. It is very important not to reinfect yourself or your partner, so keep towels and clothes separate while you have an attack. For further information on herpes treatment and support, see the Resource section.

Wart virus. At present there is a great deal of debate about whether the wart virus is involved in the development of cervical cancer. Whatever the conclusions of this debate, if you have genital warts, this is a good time to get them treated. Unfortunately for us and our partners, conventional treatment for genital warts can be lengthy and painful. One doctor suggested to me that the treatment may actually be more traumatic than the symptoms! Furthermore, many doctors are so convinced of the unlikelihood of infection that they do not even suggest that both partners be treated. If you do want treatment, however, there are a variety of remedies available and what you are offered will depend on where you attend and what your condition is: creams and antibiotics are a possibility, while another treatment uses chemicals to burn away the warts, a process which takes two to three weeks. In cauterization the warts are destroyed by the application of heat or liquid nitrogen and this is usually done under anaesthetic. If you can have a local anaesthetic, do so, but some warts can be so deep inside the vagina that you need to have a general anaesthetic for treatment. Laser treatment also destroys cervical warts, and a further possibility is to have them removed surgically. There is a new experimental drug called Immunovir which is currently being tested to support the other methods; as yet there are no positive results.

One suggested self-treatment for warts is a homoeopathic remedy, Thuja, 6 potency, tablets taken regularly over a period of four to six weeks. Thuja tincture can also be painted on the warts. A good homoeopathic chemist can supply both and advise you on usage.

For further information and support, see the Resource section.

Treating cervical ectropian

Cervical ectropian (erosion) itself is not harmful, and many doctors don't think it necessary to treat it. If you have bleeding or discharge, or have an abnormal smear, then this indicates that treatment is needed. Orthodox treatment for CIN which involves burning or freezing will do this, but if you are not having this, perhaps because you are coming back for a repeat smear, you or your doctor might decide what it is worth treating any discharge with sulfa cream which is inserted in the vagina. Remember that if the condition is harmless – that is if you get a negative result on your smear – it is usually accepted that there is no need to treat it.

Complementary medicine

There are many forms of complementary medicine. The practitioners involved work mostly outside the National Health Service and you have to pay to consult them. There is also the problem of standards, for in some areas of medicine anyone can set up as a practitioner, even without training.

Some women I spoke to reported negative experiences with complementary treatments: 'I wasn't all that convinced by it.' (Emma); while some reported positive experiences: 'My homeopath was marvellous and very supportive of my decision to have laser treatment.' (Jane G.).

The Institute of Complementary Medicine and the organization New Approaches to Cancer both offer guidelines to recommended practitioners. It is worth contacting them if you want to step outside mainstream medicine.

Most of these complementary approaches do not attempt to cure your condition, be it an infection, CIN, or cancer, and will only aim to improve your general health. Most of them suggest you use their services alongside the treatment suggested by your consultant.

Some useful complementary approaches are these:

Reflexology. Your current state of health can be revealed by an examination of your feet. Foot massage can stimulate your immune system to help you fight disease.

Iridology. The iris of the eye is studied and your current general health diagnosed. Practitioners usually offer no treatment but will probably make some recommendations about your diet and lifestyle.

Massage. There are nearly as many forms of massage as there are bodies to be massaged. Some masseurs claim to heal by touch, others to stimulate energy centres in the body so that your immune system works harder. As long as you feel comfortable with the masseur, just being relaxed will strengthen you.

Meditation. Again, there are many schools. If you feel that you are stressed and need to relax, this can be helpful. You don't always need to take a philosophy on board in order to do it. Autogenic training, a 'Westernized' form of meditation, also concentrates on deep relaxation and the repetition of a calming phrase.

Dietary therapies. Alterations to your diet can help get rid of harmful waste products and boost your immune system. Beware of too strict a diet, because it can lower your energy reserves.

Acupuncture. Pressure and needle-puncture are used to release energy along 'channels' in the body. Acupuncturists sometimes offer advice on life-styles too.

Homoeopathy. The purpose is to build health rather than to treat symptoms. One homoeopath I spoke to said he would not treat cervical conditions directly; another said he would only treat any bruising or emotional upset caused by orthodox treatment.

Visualization. Some therapists believe that by visualizing the disease, you can control it. Work done with cancer patients by the Simontons in the USA over the last decade is now famous, although the Simontons themselves are rethinking their approach.

Emotional therapies. Co-counselling provides a self-help tool to release emotion safely (and cheaply). If you feel that your recovery would be helped by being able to express your emotions more fully, this may be for you. Other forms of psychotherapy and counselling usually involve working under the guidance of another person to build your mental and emotional resources and resolve past traumas in your life. They usually entail detailed change of your ways of thinking, and might therefore be both too long-term and too expensive to consider. Some short-term therapies, such as Neuro-Linguistic Programming have a good record of quick and effective work with illness.

The Bristol Cancer Help Centre provides a rounded approach to cancer care based on a variety of alternative methods. You can spend a day or a week there, depending on your needs, learning about some of the approaches mentioned here. Bristol will accept patients who have CIN and one of them, Jane Faulkwhynes, has written a moving account of how the Help Centre helped her, which is listed in the Resources section of this book. The main direction of the treatment, however, is towards the cancer sufferer. The Bristol service is private and quite costly, and recently the Centre has been criticized for its negative effect on the disease. However, the research on which the criticism was based was retracted, and medical practitioners of all kinds agree that in terms of improving the quality of life, the Centre's work is highly effective – kind, supportive and professional. Many of its patients report long-term improvement, and visiting the Centre may well change your life for the better.

The above notes on approaches are very brief: if you want further information, contact one of the referral organizations mentioned in the Resource section of this book.

Alternative approaches – yes or no?

As to the question of whether to try any of the approaches mentioned in this chapter, there are two issues to consider: first you need to decide whether to try them, and then you need to decide whether to try to cure yourself through them. The first issue seems pretty clear cut – unless you overdose on vitamins or choose a totally incompetent therapist, you are unlikely to do yourself any harm by attempting the alternative methods. Some of them – like taking exercise or practising relaxation – can immeasurably improve the quality of your life; you might find, as some women did, that having a positive smear was the starting point of a healthier, happier lifestyle. And, increasingly, even the most stringent medical research is showing that alternative approaches do have the potential to give positive results.

To rely on these approaches alone to cure you is an altogether different matter. In this case you have to consider how serious your condition is, how much time you have, and how important it is to you to be treated by conventional methods. Here a useful guideline seems to be that mentioned earlier – if you have time between diagnosis and orthodox treatment, use it, and you may well heal yourself. If you have no time, then think carefully before you say no to orthodox methods, because they may well offer a totally effective cure.

6   Which treatment – orthodox ways

' They don't usually let you
choose . . . I just kept going
until they did. '
(Lily)

We look now at the treatments you can expect to be offered in a hospital. They all involve removing the abnormal cells in some way–by burning, freezing or cutting.

As mentioned before, there is a general disadvantage in all of these; they damage the body and create distress. 'Having third degree burns on your cervix takes a bit of getting over,' as one woman put it. Also, some of the treatments involved have to be administered under general anaesthetic, which carries its own risks. Jane G., a singer, refused to have a cone biopsy because she didn't want to have a general anaesthetic, since it involves the insertion into the throat of a ventilation tube. She changed doctors and received laser treatment, which in her case cleared the abnormal cells and didn't entail a general anaesthetic. Although it is very rare to have a positive smear during pregnancy, if you do, it is particularly important to think through the alternatives when you have two lives to look after.

You should remember that although doctors usually know their job, they also have their likes and dislikes. One consultant will favour freezing, another surgery, while a third may be in the habit of using loop diathermy. They deal with hundreds of women a week and develop patterns of treatment. You can suggest a more informed alternative based on the needs of your life once you know what options are available.

You can then perhaps negotiate with your doctor to have a different form of treatment, or change doctors to get what you want. But if two doctors in a row say that you really must have one particular form of treatment, think very carefully before you argue. One may be biased, but two is more than a coincidence.

Negotiating treatment with the doctor

When will you discuss treatment with your doctor? It will almost certainly be when the consultant diagnoses you, after the colposcopy or when the results of the biopsy or cone biopsy come back. The doctor will tell you what s/he wants to do (and when). So it is wise when going for your diagnosis to be prepared to discuss treatment at the same time. You might react strongly to your doctor's suggestions of treatment, just as you can react strongly to her/his diagnosis. Everything suggested in the chapters on examination and diagnosis applies here too; you do have the right to discuss treatment with your consultant, even if you don't get the response you want.

Whatever you feel, you will probably want to begin by asking your doctor some questions, and these are some of the questions that women I talked to asked:

> *Do you think I need treatment? If not, why not?*
> *What treatment do you think would be best for me?*
> *Why are you choosing this sort of treatment?*
> *When will this treatment happen? Now? How long will I have to wait?*
> *What will be the after effects of this treatment (on my ability to have children, make love, etc)?*
> *Will my treatment mean my changing methods of contraception (will I have to have my IUCD removed)?*
> *What would be the position if I wanted to have . . . (any form of treatment other than the one the doctor has mentioned)?*
> *Why would you not recommend this?*
> *I am concerned about these things; could I talk them through with you?*
> *When would you treat me?*
> *Will I be an outpatient? (If so, when, for how long?)*
> *Will I be an inpatient? (If so, when, for how long?)*

Discussing these things will give you some idea of the way the consultant is thinking. His/her answers may satisfy you and make you feel happier about what is happening. The final few questions will also give you an idea of that particular hospital's waiting list, and the length of your own treatment (vital points when arranging child care).

If CIN1 has been diagnosed, you may be offered treatment,

or you may also be offered the possibility of repeat smears, in order to check and monitor your condition. Doctors themselves are divided on this, pointing out that on the one hand, rushing in with treatment is not a good thing to do, and on the other hand that monitoring may be more stressful for you, as well as more expensive and time-consuming for them. The choice, ultimately, is yours. You may choose to be treated; one doctor I spoke to reported that her patients overwhelmingly opted for this solution, to get the situation over and done with. You may, however, feel that you would prefer to build your own health and try to recover from your condition alone, with the added reassurance that any possible development of the disease will be watched for. If you do choose this option, you must remember that non-treatment and monitoring must go hand in hand; it is very unwise to refuse treatment and then simply disappear into the woodwork, neglecting to return for a check-up. You may get better; if you put into practice the suggestions in Chapter 5 about building health, you may have a good chance of recovering from CIN1 by yourself. But you may get worse, and you need regular smears, at three-monthly intervals if necessary, to check exactly what is happening to your body.

Secondly, you may be offered the total opposite of postponement–treatment there and then, on the spot. This will depend on the hospital you attend, though remember that whatever their usual approach, you have the right to choose to be treated later. Postponed treatment has its drawbacks. You can end up worrying in the interval between diagnosis and cure. You can get panicky before the big day. Instant treatment has the advantage of being a solution that is so quickly offered, you have no time to get upset about the problem. 'You can get it over and done with . . . and then it's done,' as one woman said. You can walk out of the clinic knowing that in all likelihood, you need not go back except for your checkup.

Equally, you may feel that the treatment you are being offered is not the right one for you. You may want to opt for another way, and if so arrange for it to be done in another hospital.

Your doctor will react in one of a number of ways. S/he may agree to what you suggest, in which case you have got what you wanted, secure in the knowledge that your doctor believes it is medically sound.

Your doctor may disagree, and refuse to do what you have suggested. If so, do not go along with his/her suggestions right away, without taking time to think. If you are concerned, go home and think through the whole issue of treatment. Talk about it with people close to you, or with professionals if you need to. Think about just what you would prefer your treatment to be. For many of us, particularly with minor conditions, the decision is easily made. If your condition is more serious, think more carefully about which option to go for.

Treatments–the options

What follows is an outline of the various treatments, what they involve and their advantages and disadvantages. You can use this to compare different treatments and as a guide to help you understand what is happening when you have your treatment. All of them are effective, and the doctor will usually choose whichever one is most suitable for you.

Outpatient treatments

Loop diathermy is a very thin hot wire that slices through the

77

cervical tissue to remove the affected areas, cutting and sealing the cut at the same time. It is used in an ever-increasing number of clinics now; its advantages seem to be its speed and the fact that the cells don't vanish, as they do with many other forms of treatment, so that the piece of tissue can be sent to the lab for analysis. You would normally have loop diathermy in the Outpatients Department and be treated in just a few minutes. Some doctors are wary of it because it can tempt them into 'zapping' the problem away and overtreating patients; you can help offset the temptation by thinking carefully before you agree to your treatment.

Laser is an infra-red beam that vaporizes abnormal cells. Over the past few years, it has been overtaken in the popularity stakes by loop diathermy. Like loop diathermy, laser treatment has few after-effects, and is quick and easy to do; its opponents argue that it takes longer and requires more skill. Despite the fact that loop diathermy is currently more used, laser is not inferior to it in treatment terms, so if your area only offers laser you are not missing out.

Cryosurgery. Liquid nitrogen is applied in order to destroy the cells. It is usually used to treat CIN1 or 2, or generalized cervical symptoms such as bleeding, and is done in Outpatients. It is cheaper than laser.

Cold coagulation. Despite its name, a heat treatment used when a condition is not so severe, or when there are symptoms such as bleeding rather than actual abnormal cells. It is done as an outpatient treatment.

Inpatient treatments

Hot wire cautery and diathermy. This heat treatment method is not used so much now as it was even a few years ago. It is used when CIN has spread far into your cervix and cannot quite be reached by other methods, and is usually done under a general anaesthetic, with you entering hospital as an inpatient.

Cone or cylinder biopsy. This is removal of a cone- (or cylinder-) shaped piece of the cervix. It is usually done under general anaesthetic, and you will probably have to spend a few days in hospital. It is used in more advanced forms of CIN, particularly when other forms of treatment cannot reach abnormal cells that have developed far up the cervix. During the operation, the surgeon will cut out the affected cells in a cone or cylinder shape (usually by knife, though sometimes using loop diathermy or laser) and if necessary will cauterize the cervix to stop it bleeding. Soluble stitches may be added and then your vagina packed with fine gauze soaked in a cream.

Cone biopsy does have some potential dangers, among them risk to your child-bearing possibilities. Jane F. happily accepted a cone biopsy without being told that it would later mean that she would be unable to give birth normally, and only discovered this, to her horror, once she was pregnant and the gynaecologist informed her she had to have a Caesarian birth. If you are offered a cone biopsy, however, there are usually good reasons for the doctor suggesting it; discuss these with him/her, and if you have particular worries about later child-bearing, mention these specifically. There may be some other treatment option, or some option that

79

involves careful stitching of the cervix after the treatment, that can avoid these later problems.

Hysterectomy is the removal of the womb, sometimes along with the ovaries and part of the vagina and lymph nodes. When cancer has spread, hysterectomy is almost always carried out, but it may also be offered if you are past child-bearing age, even if your condition is not very serious. So check carefully what your options are before agreeing to the operation. It takes several days in hospital and weeks of recovery, and you must also consider the emotional effects of losing your womb. However, if the cancer is truly massive, then hysterectomy may be the best option.

Radiotherapy. Radiation treatment used to kill cancer, or to remove any last traces of cancer after a hysterectomy. The treatment can consist of daily doses under a machine for several weeks, or in the vagina for twenty-four hours. There are side effects, though these are often over-dramatized. It is usually only recommended when cancer is present and you need it in order to survive.

Chemotherapy. Injected drugs are used along with surgery. This is rarely used with cervical conditions. It has all the effects (and most of the side effects) of radiotherapy.

Treatment choice–outpatients

Nowadays, more and more treatments are being done as outpatient options: if you are to have loop diathermy, laser treatment, cold coagulation or cryosurgery, you will almost certainly be seen in the Outpatients Department. Some of the women I talked to had gone into hospital overnight for these treatments, because for one reason or another they had needed a general anaesthetic, but usually they are a one-day affair.

When having outpatients treatment, prepare well. You will be asked to bring a friend or partner. You may want to read over the comments in the chapters on Examination and Building Your Own Support System to help you think through the issues surrounding this. All the things I said there apply again. Also remember to book child care or time off from work–and to arrange your appointment so that it doesn't clash with your period.

If you have an IUCD, you may have been told that it has to be removed during your treatment. You will therefore need to start using another method of contraception, and this may entail some thinking ahead–for example if you want to start taking the Pill.

Take with you your own sanitary towel and perhaps some pain-killers in case you need them. One woman reported taking a homoeopathic liquid called The Rescue Remedy (for shock and trauma) immediately after her treatment, and said she felt much better within minutes.

At the hospital

After you have reached the hospital and are checked in and waiting, try preparing for what is going to happen by relaxing. This may sound difficult, for you are facing an operation, even though it is minor. But the more you relax, the less of a jolt to your system the treatment will be. As mentioned before, it is also good to give and receive support with other women in the waiting-room.

81

You may be offered counselling before your treatment. This possibility is, I am glad to say, being given to more and more women in clinics throughout the country now that medical professionals have become aware of the distress they can suffer before and after treatment–though unfortunately, as yet, the funding is not available to allow every clinic to have a counsellor. Although you may well have already confided your worries to your friends or partner (see Part 3 of this book), nevertheless, it can be good to talk to a professional. You don't have to. If you feel that you have no need to talk to anyone, that's fine. But if you do need to express some of your problems–or perhaps talk about sexual fears that you find it hard to discuss with anyone else–then a counsellor will be able to offer support and a listening ear.

After seeing the counsellor, you will probably go straight to the treatment room. This will be very similar to the room in which you initially had your examination. Most hospitals nowadays allow you to bring your friend or partner in with you, so that you have someone to hold your hand. If your hospital doesn't suggest your friend comes in with you, mention it anyway; they might say yes if you ask.

Remembering as always to take your briefs with you, you then lie down on an examination couch with your legs on supports as before. It is at this point that your IUCD, if you have one, will be removed. This can come as a great shock if you are not expecting it: 'Naughty that, not telling you,' was Rosemary's comment. Some consultants will replace your IUCD after treatment, if they are confident that this will not increase your risk of infection.

Treatment

Whichever outpatient treatment you are having–loop diathermy, laser, cold coagulation, or cryosurgery–the doctor will as usual place a speculum in your vagina and open it. Then s/he will probably give you a local anaesthetic, which is an injection into your cervix; some women complained that this was actually the most painful part of the whole process! (For cryosurgery, or for very minor treatment, a local anaesthetic is usually not necessary.) Next, as the anaesthetic begins to take effect, the consultant will dab solution on your cervix as before, to show up the abnormal areas.

Then s/he will position the treatment equipment at the entrance to your vagina, and if you are having loop diathermy, you will also have a sticky pad put on your leg, to earth the equipment. You probably won't see the machinery as you will be lying flat, although you may hear it; if you are having loop

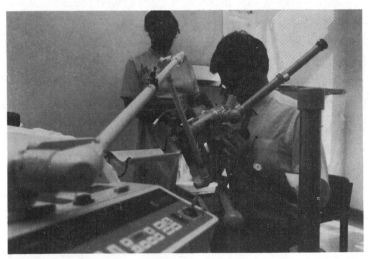

Figure 8 **Colposcopy and laser use**

83

diathermy or laser treatment, it 'makes a noise like a Hoover' as Julia said. With heat-based treatments, there may be a burning smell, which can be quite off-putting if you are not expecting it. In fact, only a microscopic amount of cells is being burned away by the treatment so it is not nearly as bad as it seems, though with laser treatment the staff may have to wear protective goggles or masks because of the constant fumes.

Does it hurt? As always, this depends on what treatment you are having, how tense you are, and how skilful the doctor is. Most clinics now will give you local anaesthetic, and if not, you can ask for it; in addition, the nurse usually stays with you, talking and often holding your hand.

How you react when it is happening also depends on many things. Mary reported that she 'lost her centre of gravity', while Emma found it 'a strong space, very relaxed . . . my partner was with me.' You can feel quite panicky, or know that at last you are being cured.

As the local anaesthetic wears off, you may need pain killers for a few hours; it is always wise to bring your own with you to the clinic so that you can take them if you need to.

Afterwards, most hospitals provide a room where you can lie down and recover after the treatment. By this time, you will have put your briefs back on, with the sanitary towel. If you can, relax and rest until you feel better, and perhaps talk to your partner or friend about how you felt and what it was like. You may not want to talk at all, but just take time to assimilate what has happened in your own way.

If possible, have a cup of something hot before going to collect the medicine that you need to take with you for afterwards. This medicine will probably be antiseptic cream, although sometimes an antibiotic is prescribed to stop your wound becoming infected.

Afterwards – physical reactions

Women react very differently to these cervical treatments. Some take them in their stride; for many there is a 'kickback', as Rosemary described it.

The physical side-effects can be quite unexpected. I found that few hospitals think to warn patients sufficiently of what to expect, probably in order not to scare them. This is important, but just as important is knowing what might happen.

All the treatments given in Outpatients have side effects of one sort or another. Many women said they felt tired and weepy; some reported faintness and dizziness. 'I tried to go shopping afterwards, but it was a mistake,' said Rosemary. If you have had a more extensive treatment you will probably need to take things very gently, go back home and rest up for a while, maybe even take a few days off work.

Another unexpected problem can be having to insert vaginal cream to heal the area that has been treated. You will need to insert an applicator containing the cream into your vagina – and this is usually best done lying on your back or your side. Some women find this difficult, others find it surprisingly funny: 'On my back, legs apart, and with one foot jammed up against the bathroom door because it doesn't have a lock on it,' was one woman's hilarious description.

You will probably have discharge whichever treatment you had: 'Smelly watery black bits,' as Julie described it; 'Bits of floating mushroom,' as Linda said. It's best to wear a sanitary towel rather than tampons for about four weeks to avoid the risk of infection. Be prepared too for bleeding which lasts much longer than you expect it to. As you leave after treatment ask your consultant for some indication of how long this bleeding might

85

last. Almost every woman I spoke to reported bleeding which was heavier or longer than she expected. If you become anxious at any time after your treatment, go, as I did, to your GP. Some hospitals provide a number to ring if you are worried–and of course if the problem is really serious, you can go to Outpatients.

The hospital will probably advise you not to have penetrative sex for a while after the treatment. Times given vary widely, according to the kind of treatment you have received and the number of abnornal cells you needed to have removed–the nicest way of putting it that I have so far read was a leaflet from the University of Dundee which advised women to start intercourse again 'just as soon as you feel comfortable with the thought'. Making love need not involve intercourse, of course–a fact many hospitals forget, thus often alienating lesbian patients–and there are many other things you can do in order to make sexual contact with your partner and receive loving comfort from him or her.

Long term side effects of these treatments seem to be very few and they shouldn't affect your ability to have children or to enjoy penetrative sex. Some women complain of spotting or light bleeding for a long time afterwards, but in general the healing is clear and clean.

Afterwards–emotional reactions

The emotional reactions to cervical treatment may be less noticeable than the physical reactions–or conversely, may last far longer. Particularly, if you have been treated at the same time as you were examined, you may find that the whole thing seems quite trivial, and is easily dealt with–or alternatively, that you feel overwhelmed by the event and take a long time to feel good about it. More than one woman commented on the feeling of being penetrated: as I mentioned before, a feeling of aversion may be stronger if penetration is not part of your natural sexual patterns, or if you have had some traumatic experience involving penetration; but even if you haven't, the contradiction between wanting to pull away and wanting to be cured may be distressing. Emma summed it up when she said, 'You feel it coming into you. You feel you need to protect yourself, yet you know you have to keep still if it is going to work.'

However, many women reported feeling elated after the treatment. They knew that the problem was now more than likely gone for ever. There can be a sense of 'triumph–I did it!' as one woman reported. Most women said they felt more negative emotions–fear, for example–before the operation, than after. Once it is over, you will quite possibly have a sense of being cured both physically and emotionally.

Treatment choice–Inpatient

You may be wary of going into hospital as an inpatient, particularly if you've never done so before. On a practical level, however, there is often very little difference between this and outpatient treatment; it just takes more time, that's all.

This section describes what the process of being an inpatient involves, particularly the process of having a general anaesthetic. Such an anaesthetic is usually used for more extensive treatment, often surgical, when a local anaesthetic just wouldn't be enough. Often, this means staying in hospital overnight, although sometimes it is possible to check in early in the morning and leave that same evening. A word of warning–if you develop a streaming cold just before the operation, don't even bother going to the hospital, as it is very unlikely they will operate. Ring them the day before, explain the situation and ask their advice.

When you arrive at the hospital, the receptionist will usually tell you which ward to report to, and when you get there a nurse will show you to a bed. The waiting, sometimes throughout that day until your operation the next morning, is often the worst. Take lots of reading (or knitting) with you and welcome visitors with open arms–you can get very bored.

The day will probably be full, however, as doctors examine you again, take a full medical history, a blood sample and check your lungs and blood pressure. Usually a junior doctor will see you to check the details, and the anaesthetist will visit you to check any problems with the anaesthetic. Occasionally the consultant who will do the operation will also call in to see you.

If you are staying overnight in hospital, don't be surprised if you can't get to sleep; you're in an unfamiliar place and probably worried about tomorrow. The nurses may offer you sleeping tablets, or you may prefer to take a herbal or calcium sleeping remedy which will leave your body feeling more alert and ready to cope with the operation; some women said they used these and found them less 'drugging' than the hospital's alternative.

You won't be allowed anything to eat on the morning of the operation, and you will be asked to bathe or shower and change into theatre clothes, a gown and cap. You'll sometimes be asked to remove your jewellery, and if you don't want to take your rings off, they can be taped to your hand.

You will be asked to sign a consent form, saying that you understand what is going to happen and agree to it. Make very sure you get this explained to you–and that you do agree. Viki refused to sign a form saying that if the surgeon found cancer cells, he could perform a hysterectomy while she was on the operating table. She preferred to wait and talk it through with him after the operation rather than agree to it in advance.

You will probably then be given a pre-medication. It is usually given to calm you down, and reduce your saliva, which can make your mouth too slippery for the anaesthetist to cope with. You can add to the calming effect of the pre-med by using your own ways of relaxing–perhaps taking deep regular breaths, or remembering a time when you were particularly calm and strong within yourself.

When you are taken from the ward, you will be checked to make sure you are the right patient–you don't want to have the wrong operation done! In the ante-room to the theatre, the anaesthetist will inject the back of your hand with an anaesthetic solution. I remember my anaesthetist had a student with him, and I lost consciousness to the refrain of 'In that vein–not that one, that one . . .'

When you wake from the anaesthetic, you will have a dull ache in your stomach, and someone will have given you a sanitary towel (although more than likely not the briefs, so it will stick to the inside of your leg in a most off-putting manner).

If you have had a cone biopsy, you may well have had your vagina stuffed with gauze. It is likely that you will be uncomfortable–'it brings water to your eyes' (Lily)–but the discomfort eases after the gauze is taken out. Sometimes you also have to have a catheter inserted to allow you to pass water.

As you wake, you will possibly be offered water to drink or ice to suck, and left to recover. This can take a few hours, or overnight, depending on the operation you've had, and you can expect to be very sleepy as a result of the drugs.

In some hospitals, women go home the same day, but in most,

they stay in another night and are discharged after the consultant has seen them the next morning. Particularly with a cone biopsy, you can be asked to stay a day or two until you feel really better. The hospital will almost certainly give you antibiotics to help the healing process, and full instructions on how and when to take these.

Afterwards–physical reactions

The after-effects of these more extensive treatments can be slightly more offputting than those of the outpatient treatments. If you do have hot wire treatment, discharge and bleeding can last a long time. I bled for five weeks, and on the fifth week, dropped a blood clot that terrified me–although I then learned from my doctor that this is perfectly normal and is caused by the scab dropping off the cervical wound. In addition, the antibiotics I was given made me nauseous all the time.

The long-term physical effects of hot wire/diathermy are usually the same as for outpatient treatments–none. The

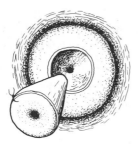
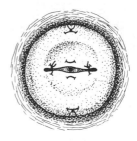

The cone removed   The raw area covered

Figure 9 **Cone biopsy. A cone-shaped wedge of tissue is removed from the cervix**

after-effects of a surgical cone biopsy are usually bleeding problems. This is why the hospital may suggest you stay in for a day or two after the operation so that if serious bleeding starts, they can treat you. You will continue to bleed for some time and may need to take it very easy while you convalesce, though Evelyn discharged herself from hospital the day after her operation and went straight to a weekend course.

It is probably quite unwise to have penetrative sex before several weeks have passed, to give your cervix time to heal–though ask your consultant about this. Bleeding might start again, or an infection take hold, and you are very vulnerable at this time. The long-term effects of a cone biopsy can vary. Rachel's cervix closed together after her operation, and she had to have a second one to open it again. If this happens, your periods may stop (although you have to check that you aren't pregnant) and this can lead to complications. There is also a slight chance–as happened to Jane F., whose story is described earlier in this chapter–that having a cone biopsy may affect your ability to have children, and that you may not find this out until many years later. If so, you may, like Jane, both feel angry and grieve.

As both hotwire/diathermy involve general anaesthetic, you may feel the after-effects of this too. It could take you days to feel really alert, depending on just how the antibiotics affect you and the amount of anaesthetic and pre-medication you've had. Remember that they are meant to slow down your nervous system and this is exactly what they do. Some women bounce straight back; some take a weekend of being sleepy and weepy before going back to work. After a cone biopsy take a few days convalesence if this is possible; your doctor will probably tell you how long to rest for.

Afterwards—emotional reactions

In some ways, inpatient operations can leave you less emotional than outpatient operations. You aren't left with the memories of having things done to you, and you don't need to cope with 'pulling yourself together' directly afterwards in order to go home.

On the other hand, these operations take a much bigger chunk out of your life. You may be out of action for a while, and you will be away from your home base at least overnight. Also, you are on your own, negotiating the hospital routine and the discomfort of the operation, without a friend or partner to hold your hand.

When you come out of hospital, try to make sure there is someone at home to be with you, at least overnight. One woman said, 'My partner picked me up from the hospital, brought me home and then went off on a golfing weekend. Even though I encouraged him to go, I still never quite forgave him.'

Expect to feel a bit odd for a while, particularly if you've had a cone biopsy and have been under general anaesthetic for longer. Take your support where you can, and give yourself time to get over things, physically and emotionally: 'I went straight from my cone biopsy off to a group of friends,' said one woman, 'and lapped up all the sympathy and looking-after I got!'

Treatment choice—radical methods

Radical treatments tend to be treatments that make us scared—hysterectomy, radiotherapy, chemotherapy. There are lots of horror stories about things that go wrong, and how awful it can all be.

Mostly these treatments are used to cure cancer—although in

the case of hysterectomy, it could be for a persistent pre-cancer or for treating other gynaecological problems at the same time.

If your doctor has said that you need to have one of these treatments, then you can choose not to have it. But as I said before, it is usually better, in these serious cases, to agree to the treatment. Supplement what is happening to you with your own ways of getting yourself better.

Build your health, physically and emotionally, and use all the resources you have–people, information, spiritual beliefs–to make the experience as positive as you can. Because this is a book about the whole experience of positive smear, and because radical treatments are called for in only a very small proportion of cases, I am only outlining what happens. At the back of the book you will find suggestions for reading matter in the form of specialist leaflets and books as well as the address of support groups and counselling services. Use them as starting points to get your own support system together.

There are two particular areas where you are likely to feel vulnerable. If you have gone from one examination to another, hoping for good news and always getting bad news, you may, like Sue did, 'feel my optimism waning'. If you know you have invasive cancer, you may be scared you are going to die. This is unlikely, but it is a fear you will naturally face, and you can find other people uneasy with it. Your partner may have emotions of his own to cope with, and relatives and friends may be unable to talk to you because they fear the worst – although Vivienne comments that on telling her parents about her hysterectomy, 'My dear Mum realized all too well what that meant and we wept in each other's arms.'

Also, the thought of losing your ability to bear children can create strong emotion for you. If you are not yet past the age where you could have children, it may make you feel sad and as if you have lost something. Vivienne commented, 'I was to be plummeted into the menopause as if it didn't matter,' and another woman said about her hysterectomy, 'it's not a form of contraception that I'd recommend.'

There are support groups in most areas of the country where you can talk to women who have had a hysterectomy, get support from them and discuss your problems. Also, it's likely that the hospital you go to will offer you some counselling both before and after your hysterectomy. 'I cried a lot in hospital,' said Diana, 'away from the children in privacy. It's my way of coping with it.'

However, one nurse I spoke to made the very valid comment that because hospitals are working so speedily to treat conditions like cervical cancer, you may well actually miss out on the counselling element: if you are rushed into an emergency 'slot' in the ward, they are so keen to treat your body that they forget about your emotions. So ask for support from staff in the hospital if you need it; if there are counselling facilities available at all, they are yours by right.

Final checks

It is likely that just before you have your treatment, your doctor will want to have a final check to see how far the cancer has spread.

One may be a kidney scan (IVU or IVP) to check that cancer has not spread to your kidneys. This is rarely the case, but if so, it does mean you are seriously ill. You will have a dye injected in a vein, probably in your arm. It goes through your bloodstream and ends up in kidneys, bladder and urethra. You may feel a slight burning, but this soon passes, and then the kidney X-ray will be taken.

Another type of scan that may be done is a Pelvic CT or CAT scan. A complete picture of your womb and the organs around it is taken by several small X-rays that are collected by computer and displayed on to a TV screen. You will be asked to drink a special liquid, a tampon will be put into your vagina, and a liquid inserted into your anus. This allows your entire pelvis to be X-rayed effectively.

Another type of scan is the ultrasound scan. For this you will first be asked to drink lots of liquid to get a full bladder. My own experience of this is that there are better ways of spending an afternoon than lying on a couch being examined while your only desire in the world is to have a pee. A gel is spread over the surface of your abdomen and then a microphone is pressed down upon it. This sends silent sound waves rippling through your full bladder. The echoes of these sound waves are collected and converted by computer to make a picture that the doctor can examine.

A final test that might be done is a lymphogram, which checks whether your lymph system has been affected. Dye is injected into your feet, and will then pass through the lymph system up to your pelvis. An X-ray shows the doctor how the dye is passing through the system, and where any problems lie. The whole process takes a few hours, and will have the interesting side effect of your skin and urine turning a green colour.

Hysterectomy

There are various kinds of hysterectomy, depending on just

95

what is being taken away. A total hysterectomy is usually
performed on women with earlier forms of cancer. This
means that both the uterus and the cervix are removed, though
not always the ovaries. In the case of younger women
especially, the ovaries are usually left intact in order to avoid
early menopausal symptoms. If more of your pelvis has been
affected by the cancer, then your lymph glands might also be
removed. Ask your consultant to explain to you exactly how
s/he has planned your operation and what s/he needs to
remove; remember that s/he has to explain the options to you
and give you the right of final veto.

Although the operation is sometimes done through the

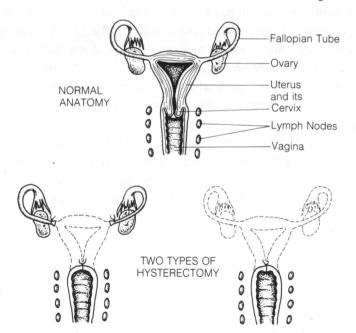

Figure 10 **The extent of total hysterectomy**

vagina, it is more commonly performed by abdominal incision, a horizontal cut being made above your pubic hair; the scar usually heals well and is almost invisible. The alternative is a downwards cut, and you should check which your surgeon is doing. Sometimes a downwards cut cannot be avoided, but if possible ask if you can have the horizontal one–it's neater.

The preparations for a hysterectomy are the same as for any of the other operations mentioned in this book, except that you will be given a suppository to empty your bowels, and a section at the top of your pubic hair will be shaved off. It does grow back!

When you go for your operation, you will usually be given the anaesthetic in the back of your hand, as described earlier. Very occasionally you will be given an epidural, which means that the anaesthetic is injected into your spinal cord. This is similar to the anaesthetic administered to women when giving birth and it numbs the whole area below the point where the injection is given. The operation itself usually takes about an hour. After your womb has been removed, the vagina is closed at the top and the abdomen stitched or clamped closed. As you wake up, you may find you are feeling sick, and your abdomen is hurting. You will have a drip attached to your arm for liquid or blood, and a catheter to drain fluids from your bladder. You will also have a drain in your pelvis and possibly one from the wound.

The recovery from hysterectomy varies from woman to woman. There is no single universal reaction, but you can expect to experience some discomfort. At first you will only be allowed sips of fluid, to make sure your system can cope as it gets back to normal. The wound drain will probably be removed within a day, and the pelvic drain in about a week. The catheter will go when you are able to cope without it – from a day or two to several days. You will be encouraged to move around to prevent blood clots.

If you have had your ovaries removed you may start to experience hot flushes, as the menopause starts. You may be offered hormone replacement therapy (HRT), to offset these symptoms. If for some reason your consultant says it would be unwise for you to have HRT, then ask him/her to explain why, and check whether instead you could have one of the other substitutes that can relieve the symptoms.

The after-effects of hysterectomy can last a while. You may have a reduced bladder capacity, and have to retrain your bladder. If you want to have penetrative sex, you may find you need to go carefully until your newly shortened vagina gets stretched again, and you may find that your natural lubrication is less than it was.

You may also feel weepy and need lots of reassurance from your partner. He/she will also be coping with his/her own emotional reaction; many of the women I talked to found that going through this thing together actually brought them closer to their partners. Try to get lots of cuddles and physical affection if you can, and give yourself and your partner time and space to discuss how you feel about what has happened.

Radiotherapy

In radiotherapy high-energy rays destroy the cancer. It can be used in a number of ways: before a hysterectomy to shrink the tumour; after a hysterectomy to destroy the last remnant of cancer cells, or 'knock it on the head' as Jane B. said; or often on its own instead of surgery. It can be used internally and externally.

The first step is to plan your treatment, and for this you'll go to the radiotherapy department for a few explanatory visits. The radiographer will do a Pelvic CT or CAT scan to find out just where the radium treatment is needed. As described on page 95 a tampon will first be placed in your vagina and a liquid put into your anus. Remember that the nurses are used to doing this, and that a little embarrassment is worth it when it is saving your life.

You usually have external radiotherapy as an outpatient and will probably have to attend hospital three or four times a week, over perhaps six weeks. The radiographer will make marks on your skin, and then position you on a couch under the machine. The treatment may take several minutes, but it usually isn't painful, 'just boring' as one woman said. You will usually be able to communicate with the nurses through an intercom, and they will be watching you on a closed circuit television to check that you are all right.

Internal radiotherapy is usually done in hospital and you will be in a room on your own; plastic applicators are placed inside your vagina and inside these are put radioactive caesium rods. You have to lie very still so that they don't move and only affect the area they are meant to heal. You should feel little pain, though taking the applicators out can be painful, and of course lying still for ages is uncomfortable. 'I got very lonely,' said one woman I talked to, as she described how visitors and nurses could not come in so that they would not be affected by the radiation.

Both of these treatments can have side effects: Sue said that she was 'very near giving up at one point; it didn't seem worth it.' Nausea, diarrhoea and a cystitis-like pain when passing water can occur and make your life very uncomfortable, and you will feel tired and weepy a lot of the time. But many hospitals give tablets to cope with all these side effects, and they do not last for ever.

Even if you haven't had a hysterectomy, radiotherapy will stop your ovaries working and you will experience menopausal symptoms, possibly including loss of desire. Again, ask for hormone replacement therapy if you want to. Just as with hysterectomy, you may feel depressed at the thought of not being able to have children–allow yourself all the support you need, and give yourself time to recover.

Chemotherapy

In chemotherapy drugs are used to destroy cancer cells. It is usually administered when the cancer has spread to various parts of your body, and is not often used for cervical cancer; its use will depend on your particular illness.

The drugs damage the cells to stop them dividing and are given over a period of time which can vary from a few weeks to several months. They are usually injected into a vein, though sometimes they may be swallowed as tablets or capsules.

They affect normal cells as well as cancer cells, and therefore have a number of side effects. You can get very tired and will need to rest a lot. You will vomit, and may have ulcers on your mouth. You won't however, with the usual form of chemotherapy used for cervical cancer, lose your hair.

As your blood cells are affected, you are vulnerable to infections, so you need to build up your general health as much as you can. If you do catch an infection, the hospital will usually treat it with antibiotics or even blood transfusions.

Final thoughts

All these radical treatments can sound horrendous but don't let things get out of proportion. If you are reading this book having just been diagnosed CIN 1 or 2, then most of this information is probably not relevant to you at all. Read about it to find out what can happen to other women, but don't panic.

If you have CIN 3, then similarly you have an excellent chance of only ever experiencing these treatments by reading about them since they are usually only used if you have invasive cancer.

If you do have to have one or more of these treatments, that is tough to handle. You will need support and you will need to be flexible and brave. But if the women I have talked to are anything to go by, you will make some meaning out of what is happening, and you will be able to look back in a few years and see it all in a new perspective. And perhaps tell other women who are going through it how you survived . . .

7   Prevention

' Now, I feel I'm doing
something to take charge ... I'm
taking control of my own health. '
(Tracey)

What do you need to do in order never to have a positive smear? Or in the case of those of us who have had one, whether we needed treatment or not, what can we do in order never to have one again?

The first step, I think, is to realize that we have a choice. There are things we can do that make us vulnerable, and there are things we can do to make us less vulnerable. We are adults now, and no one is going to shout at us if we do some of the 'wrong' things and miss out some of the 'right' things. Admittedly some of the Government warnings and some of the quoted medical professionals speak to us like children, telling us that if we aren't good little girls, the bogyman will come and get us. Some of them also tell us that it is our fault that the bogyman is on the loose at all.

We do still have a choice. If we choose, we can avoid positive smears, we can go some way to avoiding cervical cancer altogether by following all the guidelines for its prevention. Or if we choose we can adopt some of them, and leave the rest to fate. If instead we smoke heavily, are on the Pill, make love unprotected with a new man every night, we are in effect stacking the odds against ourselves, and that is our choice.

Prevention possibilities

Build your health

Almost anything you do to build your health will give you a better chance of not developing cervical conditions. Many infections, which are breeding grounds for CIN, develop when we are run down. CIN and cancer can advance more rapidly if our immune systems are low and not working properly. A body that is fighting the debilitating effects of being overweight, of foods that stimulate allergies, or under-exercised heart and lungs, will be less able to cope with fighting off illness than a body that is running like a well-tuned engine.

The following are some guidelines and things to think about when deciding how to build your health and strengthen your immune system.

Food. A good diet is essential to health. 'We cut out fat and sugar, and we eat salads, fish and chicken.' (Sue). Eating unrefined foods such as whole grains will give you a healthier, high-fibre diet. Fresh fruit and vegetables contain more vitamins than canned or frozen.

Avoid any foods that you feel you are allergic to. Common

allergies are to coffee, tea, wheat and dairy products, so if you suspect you have a bad reaction to any of these, try cutting them out of your diet and re-introducing them one at a time. Foods that contain flavourings and colourings, or have been sprayed with pesticide can affect you too, so check pre-packed foods for E numbers and avoid them if you can.

Don't diet constantly. In fact, try not to diet at all; denying your body essential nutrients can do more harm than good. Instead, try to have a balanced diet. Eat only when you are hungry, and stop immediately you feel the first signs of fullness – remember that your stomach is only the size of a closed fist, so a heaped plateful is usually far too much. Burn off excess calories, as well as reducing your chances of heart disease, through regular exercise. If you have an eating problem, such as anorexia nervosa or bulimia, or even suspect that you have, ask your GP to refer you for expert help immediately.

Drugs. Limit your alcohol intake. Fourteen units of alcohol is the maximum you should drink each week, with one unit being a glass of wine or spirits, a half-pint of ordinary beer or a quarter pint of extra-strength beer. So try not to take more than two or three standard drinks two or three times a week, and keep the other days alcohol free. If you do overdo it and get drunk, take a break from alcohol over the next week or so, to give your body a chance to recover. Keep clear of all kinds of hard drugs, and if you can, avoid using soft drugs, pain-killers or tranquillizers. Obviously if you have been prescribed them by your doctor you should first check with him/her that stopping them will be all right.

Vitamins. Find good prolonged-release nutrition multivitamin and mineral tablets to take each day. Make sure you take enough vitamin C (particularly if you smoke), B vitamins (particularly if you are on the Pill), and vitamin A. Don't, however, overdose on vitamins: too much of some can stress your system.

Exercise. Take regular exercise. The best is a combination of regular and vigorous exercise during each week. This could include some regular gentle exercise to build stamina, and two or three bouts of vigorous exercise to get your heart and lungs working. A regular walk to work, an exercise class and a swimming session would be ideal. Don't try to exercise if you hate it—but find some sort of exercise (dance, competitive games, running) that you can get enthusiastic about. If you get bored exercising, buy a personal stereo—or find a companion.

Check-ups. Keep an eye out yourself for any changes in your body's workings—sudden tiredness, alteration in urine or faeces, odd bumps or moles. There is currently some controversy about whether rigorous monthly breast checks, using your fingers to check for lumps, are effective; but it is still worthwhile being aware, as you look in the mirror or touch yourself in the bath, of any changes in your breasts, whatever they may be.

Mental health. Many studies have shown that attitude and emotional state have a deep impact on our health. Begin by making sure that you are not mentally stressed; take some time each day to relax and allow yourself to assimilate what you have done and seen. Meditation, stress-reduction techniques, yoga, relaxation tapes or simply sitting and thinking will do. If you find yourself feeling unhappy or depressed in a long-term way, whether this is triggered by a life event such as bereavement or whether it simply creeps up on you for no reason at all, then get support. Feeling low is not something you need to accept; you can do something about it. Contact friends, make plans, get out more. Go to a counsellor, which is not a sign you are mentally ill, but a sign that you are sane enough to want to get well. If your mind and emotions are on the up, your body will be far more able to fight off disease.

Stop smoking

In my parents' day, smoking was the fashionable thing to do. Nowadays, it is distinctly unfashionable. Very few of the women I spoke to smoked. One gave up immediately after her hysterectomy. Only a few chain-smoked their way through the interview.

Stopping smoking will decrease your risk of getting cervical cancer – that is a fact. It will also increase your ability to run, play, work, make love – and breathe. Your skin will look better and you will be less likely to die of heart and lung disease. But if you do smoke, none of this may matter. Even the thought of cervical cancer can seem a long way away while the thought of the next cigarette is all-attractive. There are ways to stop smoking, although to date no one has discovered one which always works for everyone. You could try one of the patent remedies available in chemists' shops. You could read one of a number of 'stop smoking' books. You could join a support group. You could examine what you get out of smoking – relaxation, social acceptance, a sense of elegance – and try getting these things in other ways. Whatever, bear in mind that

Positive Smear

you are giving up an addiction, and that it may be a challenge; don't mentally beat yourself up if you slip, and don't make a lapse the excuse for going back to smoking full-time.

You could also try counselling to help you give up. Many counsellors offer stop-smoking cures, and you could even try hypnotherapy, in which your subconscious mind is invited to help you find other things to do rather than smoke.

It could be that one of these methods works for you. Perhaps, like one of the women I spoke to, you are able to 'stop just like that' once you realize that to continue could lead to another positive smear.

Cleanliness

Keeping clean is one obvious way to minimize the risk of developing cervical cancer. Washing genitals, particularly before making love, is both sensible and can be extremely erotic if you do it together. And if you or your partner live or work in a 'dirty' area, where chemicals, diesel fuel, asbestos or mining dirt is in the air, then it is absolutely essential. Some sources also say that neither of you should use talcum powder on your genitals, and that perfumed tampons, douches and wipes should also be avoided.

In a more general sense, fight for better working and living conditions–showers at work, bathrooms and washing machines in the home–for yourself, your partner and for other women at risk.

Coming off the Pill

As I explain in the chapter on Causes, there is some evidence

108

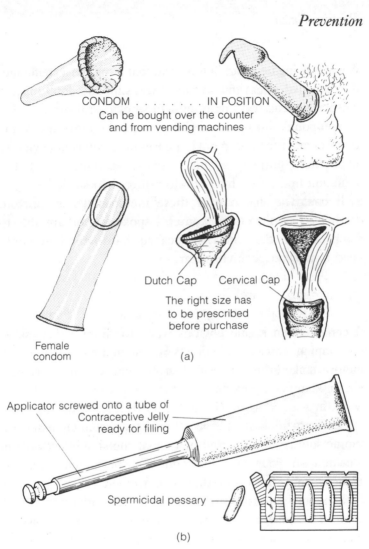

CONDOM . . . . IN POSITION
Can be bought over the counter
and from vending machines

Dutch Cap   Cervical Cap

The right size has
to be prescribed
before purchase

Female
condom

(a)

Applicator screwed onto a tube of
Contraceptive Jelly
ready for filling

Spermicidal pessary

(b)

Figure 11a **Barrier contraceptive methods. You will notice that only the condom gives complete protection against the transmission of viruses**

Figure 11b **These are often used in conjunction with barrier contraceptive methods**

109

to suggest that taking the contraceptive pill increases the likelihood of abnormal cervical conditions[3]. Changing to another method of contraception will reduce this risk. The main options are: natural birth control, IUCD, barrier methods such as the cap or the condom, or, coming soon, the female condom.

Natural birth control needs a lot of knowledge and dedication to make it work, but its advantages are that it doesn't involve the insertion of a foreign body into your cervix, as the IUCD does, or chemicals in your vagina, as some barrier methods do. However, it is notoriously unreliable (18 – 24 per cent failure rate) and demands a great deal of self- (and partner-) control.

The IUCD allows for spontaneity, but is not 100 per cent fail-safe and does make you vulnerable to infection (I speak as one who knows . . .). If you have just had treatment for a positive smear, you will know that you need to have the IUCD removed during treatment, and may have to wait a while for it to be re-inserted.

Barrier methods are less spontaneous than the Pill, but have the advantage of protecting you from possible infections. If you are in a stable heterosexual relationship and are taking the Pill, but would like to change to a barrier method, you need to discuss this first with your partner. He may feel that this will spoil the spontaneity of making love or he may be worried about the increased possibility of your becoming pregnant. If you want him to wear a condom he may feel threatened or that he is being asked to take too much responsibility.

If you are not in a regular relationship, then you will have to learn how to explain to a new partner that you are using a method of contraception that involves some forethought.

Barrier methods of contraception

At the time of going to press, the evidence linking sexual experience and cervical cancer is unclear. In particular, as mentioned in the section of this book on Causes, there is conflicting evidence of the link between the wart virus and cervical conditions.

However, many heterosexual women are choosing to use barrier contraception, to protect themselves against a possible 'cancer trigger' from their partner. This is true even when a woman has only one partner, and has been with him for many years: 'I won't have sex without a condom now, and I'm sure throughout my life I'll always use one.' (Julie). It is unclear from the evidence whether these women are being extremely wise or far too panicky. Current media publicity suggests the former. Several doctors I spoke to also said that women were wise to protect themselves. 'In the United States, they recommend all positive smear patients to use barrier contraception for life,' said one consultant. Also, a study in treating CIN conditions by using barrier methods showed remarkable effectiveness (see page 64).

Conversely, some doctors believe, and have told patients, that there is only a coincidential link between making love unprotected and developing cervical conditions, and that there are so many other possible things that could trigger CIN that using barrier contraception may be irrelevant. Few doctors suggested to women I interviewed that they should use barrier methods of contraception as a way of preventing further development of CIN.

At the same time many doctors indicated that once a woman has received treatment for CIN, any viruses may well be effectively removed. 'There was evidence of the wart virus,' Anna was told, 'but it will have gone now.' Although we know that the virus can remain in the folds of the vagina, these doctors were confident enough of the unlikelihood of its precipitating cervical abnormality and so did not suggest using barrier contraception.

The nearest to common sense I seemed to get is this: especially in this AIDS age, you will obviously want to protect yourself from all infections and viruses, whether or not they are relevant to cervical cancer. So unless you and your partner show no evidence of any virus, have known each other for a while, and both only sleep with each other, you will probably choose barrier methods of contraception. If you do have a long-term relationship, and are confident both of each other's fidelity and of each other's health, you will probably choose otherwise. There may, of course, be factors other than infections and viruses that can cause you cervical problems—for example your partner's sperm—but you may want to take that risk.

Remember too that viruses are not only present when symptoms show—they can develop or remain, and you will have to take a decision whether to chance this or not. Even if you have never had a virus, you could have contracted one from your last sexual partner. You can certainly check—if your partner is willing and doesn't mind the discomfort—that he is not infected with the wart virus, by asking him to dab a mild vinegar and water solution over his penis. Infected areas will show up white when examined with a magnifying glass. This won't, of course, give you information about whether you yourself are clear of the virus.

If you are not clear of viruses and infections, or your partner is not clear or will not go to be checked, then you can protect yourself by using a barrier method. If you have no regular partner, you could use a barrier method until you are sure that each partner is not carrying any virus. Asking a new partner to go for a check-up can be embarrassing, but once you are sure you have a steady relationship, it may be worthwhile.

A last, intriguing thought: Mary reports going on a course for safer sex which included the erotic possibilities of inserting caps and putting on condoms. A lovely idea—could your evening institute run a course like that . . .?

Not having penetrative sex

Two of the women I spoke to had done this. Hilda said: 'If sex was going to cause that many problems, I decided I wouldn't have any more relationships . . . until I'd done what I wanted to in my career.'

This might be a real possibility for you, particularly if as a result of your positive smear experience you are feeling bitter about your partner, or about men in general. Remember though that abnormal cervical conditions may result from a number of factors, and not making love that involves penetration does not mean that your safety is guaranteed.

It is also significant that some media coverage of the cervical cancer problem hints that until women stop making love then they will continue to get cervical cancer. I hope no woman will fall for this victim-blame by ceasing to make love out of guilt.

Screening

Interestingly, when newspaper headlines or medical journals

113

talk about prevention, they usually mean screening–in other words, the smear test or cervicography.

It seems strange to me to call it prevention when what is happening is merely diagnosis–a bit like a dentist suggesting that you come for regular check-ups but don't bother to clean your teeth. The argument is that if we call screening prevention, then women will feel they are involved and are taking charge–and this is a good point. But I would prefer to see women taking charge at a much earlier stage in the process. Much of the screening would be rendered unnecessary if we took care of the primary prevention.

There is currently a medical movement recommending that routine screening be stopped, or at any rate limited[4-6]. Doctors point out that the rates of cervical cancer in some countries have not gone down a great deal since screening was introduced, and that in other countries, the rates have dropped even though there is no nationwide screening programme. In addition, they say, the trauma of a smear test, the possibility of over-treatment, and the emotional effects of a positive result actually outweigh the good that a screening programme does. Opponents point out that, whether or not in general terms screening reduces a cancer statistic, for the woman whose health is preserved by a smear test, the benefits win every time.

What does this mean for you? While screening does not alter the statistics, and certainly does not prevent, only diagnose, it is certainly worth using it as a tool in your own health care. *Remember that the occurrence of invasive cancer in women who are regularly screened is practically zero.*

So should you go for screening? Of course if you are on the Pill, if you smoke, if you are about to get pregnant, if you have symptoms, you should make a special effort. But over and beyond this all women should have regular screening. There is a temptation to think that if you are a lesbian woman, or if you are celibate, then you are safe—yet women in both these categories have been known to develop CIN and cervical cancer; there are many more possible promoters of these conditions than simply heterosexual contact. There is a temptation to think that because you are older, and your sex life may have ceased, then you are safe—but there are more examples of cervical cancer in the older age group than the younger, simply because older women tend to avoid screening. And there is a temptation to postpone the test—maybe through embarrassment, maybe through fear of the result. But the fact remains that we have in our hands a powerful weapon to spot potential cancer before it starts—and we should use it.

Happily nowadays, we are often encouraged to do so by regular reminders from our GP or local clinic who, under the new government contract, are given incentives to screen all women between the ages of 25 (20 in Scotland) and 64 (60 in Scotland) every five years. (If you have had previous problems, you will be offered one more regularly—if you yourself feel you need a more regular smear, then you will have to demand one from your doctor, or pay for it privately.)

Nationwide screening recall is, of course, a great step forward. But there is also an issue here of autonomy: if you refuse your smear, you may well be pressured by your doctor, who needs to 'get the rates up' and thus claim his or her extra funding. I do worry that such a programme, whilst in theory offering women a wonderful chance to prevent cancer, is in fact also taking the preventative decision out of their hands. Why not inform women of what they can do, not just by screening, but also through the other actions mentioned in this chapter, and then support them in helping themselves, rather than by laying down a mandatory screening programme, haranguing them to attend it, and then asking them to be grateful that the system has done them a favour?

Future possibilities

As this book goes to press, there are a number of medical trials in progress which explore other options for cervical cancer prevention. None of them are available to the public, but all of them are exciting possibilities.

An Australian study has developed a cerviprobe[7], which sends pulses to tissues around the cervix, picks up the return signals and transforms them into a computer picture. The computer makes a noise if the tissues touched are pre-cancerous or cancerous. As this book goes to press, however, the method is still at research stage. A new British way of measuring forms of DNA in cervical cells may offer us a more accurate way of spotting CIN or carcinoma, thus avoiding the error factor that is so worrying in normal smear tests.

In the United Kingdom, two different studies are exploring the possibility of a cervical cancer vaccine[8]. The Cambridge study wants to use this not only to treat women with CIN, to prevent this condition developing, but also to vaccinate teenage boys and girls, to stop the problem from ever starting.

Finally, research[9] which seems to have established a link between high levels of the wart virus HPV 16 and the possibility of CIN 3 for women who have mild dyskariosis also suggests that the test they used to detect HPV 16 in this study could be developed for general use. Then, a mild grade of dyskariosis spotted on a smear test could be further checked for the wart virus: if none were found, then further investigation could probably be avoided.

What now?

We don't really know what causes cervical cancer, and until we do there can be no foolproof prevention. In the meantime, there are ways we can make ourselves less vulnerable. There are ways we can decrease the odds.

A final very positive thought is that if you have had an abnormal smear, and through treatment have had your condition cured, then you are in the lowest possible risk bracket in the future. Once you have then had a clear result, you have a much lower than average chance of getting the condition again. You are in fact in a better position than women who have never had a positive smear.

And if having a positive smear is the mechanism by which we stop and think about our health, and choose a healthier life style, then in fact for some women, it is worth it. 'Before, I used to feel ill a lot,' said Anna. 'Now, things are going really well.'

2   the facts

8   What are the facts?

‘ I was sure the more I knew and
understood, the better I'd be. ’
(Linda)

Knowledge is power. Knowing what is happening to you makes you far less vulnerable, and means that you can cope with what is going on. Understanding the facts and knowing what you are talking about when speaking to a doctor means that you can address her/him with authority.

There is a danger. If you know some things and not others, you can get frightened. Janet 'panicked at a section in a book about lymph involvement in cancer patients – and I'd only just got my smear test result . . .' Equally, some recent studies have shown that not all of us want, or are at ease with, a flood of information – it can make us worry even more. So if you feel you do not want to know, then respect that feeling and don't seek out information unnecessarily, and if you want the facts, get them in a balanced way, not one that makes you panic.

Where to get information

You may need a large dictionary to help with the medical
terms, but nevertheless there are ways of getting both specific
and general information about what is happening!

First, ask your own doctor, and when the time comes, the
consultant. They are experts on the disease, even though they
are not always expert at explaining things. Remember that a
book will give you generalities – only your own doctor can
discuss your particular case with you. Elsewhere in this book
we suggest specific questions you might want to ask. Some
medical professionals don't realize that women need to know
what is happening and many women spoke of having to ask
their doctors repeatedly for general information about cervical
conditions, and specific information about their condition in
particular. 'Tell women to sit there until they get the
information,' recommended Julia – and this is exactly what
many women had to do.

The hospital you go to will very likely have its own
information leaflets setting out the relevant facts in simple
language. These are often written by staff or ex-patients who
have been through it all themselves. They rarely address
emotional issues; their strength is the clear presentation of
facts. If your hospital hasn't got a leaflet, suggest they get some
copies of the excellent ones published by Women's Health
(address in Resource Section of this book) – or even offer to
write them yourself! Diana did: 'I ended up preparing leaflets
for them.'

While waiting to see the doctor and the specialist though,
you can gain a lot of useful background knowledge. Many of
the women I spoke to got up at some point during our

conversation and said 'I'll just go and get the file . . .' The idea of The File, into which you put all the information you are gathering, became a catch phrase. So start your own 'File'!

Try reading some of the leaflets and books mentioned in the Resource section at the back of this book. There are also some videos that you can buy, and though they are not cheap, maybe your local FPC would be persuaded to pay the cost if you ran a women's evening to show them. The better alternative is usually to hire. See the Resource section for details.

You can also keep an eye open for news of recent developments on the cervical cancer front in newspapers, magazines and on the television and radio. 'Once you know about it, you pick up little snippets from everywhere,' (Rosemary). But be prepared for biased reporting. It isn't news to say: 'Most women need minor treatment after a positive smear.' It is news to dwell on the once-a-decade horror story.

A final way to gain knowledge is to talk to other women. But remember that many of them, like you, will be scared and upset, and their stories will reflect this and stress the unhappy bits. That said, women supporting women by passing on accounts of their own condition is probably one of the best kinds of information you will get. It is, after all, based on first-hand experience.

In this book, I am aiming only to give the basics. As one woman said: 'Simple, everyday language please; I'm not in the mood for long words.' If you want more detailed information, a more medically-based guide to cervical cancer will help you.

The basics

Your reproductive system

Your womb is nestled inside your pelvis for comfort and protection. On either side of it lie the ovaries which hold the eggs. The base of the womb situated at the top of the vagina, is called the cervix. After penetrative sex, your partner's sperm travels from the vagina through a small opening in the cervix, up the cervical canal, and into the womb. Every month during your period, the lining of the womb detaches itself and flows down the cervical canal, through the cervix and into the vagina.

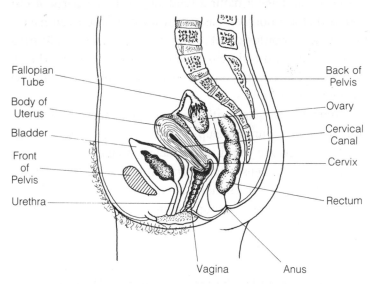

Figure 12 **Your reproductive system**

Various other organs are situated around the womb. Most, like the kidneys and bladder, are responsible for getting rid of waste products from your body. Some, like the lymph glands, protect your body against disease.

The cervix is fairly well protected by being inside your body, but since it comes into contact with the outside environment it is also quite vulnerable.

Finding out about the cervix

It's still quite rare for a woman to feel comfortable about exploring the sexual parts of her body. We don't have the advantages that men do, with 'everything on the outside'!

But we do have a natural tendency to touch parts of our bodies that are not well – as you will know when you have a mouth ulcer or bitten cheek, and your tongue inexorably drifts back to it time and again. So it is totally natural to want to begin to come to terms with your cervix by exploring it and finding out more about it.

If you want to, stand with one foot on a chair, or lie flat on your back with your knees up. Put your finger carefully inside your vagina. (Wash your hands first, and make sure your nails are short in case you scratch yourself.) Feel inside your vagina to the end; the cervix is there. Some women describe it as a 'dome shape', a 'lump', a 'bump with a dip in it'. It feels firmer than the soft walls of the vagina, and as one woman said: 'Once you've found it, you'll know . . .'

Those of us who use the cap, which involves checking that the cervix is covered each time we put it in, will be used to this. The rest of us may take some time to find out which is cervix and which is the rest of our vagina. Remember too that the

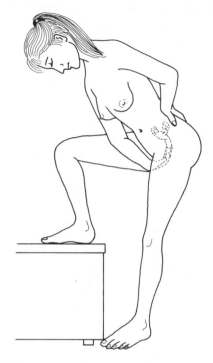

Figure 13 **Exploring your vagina and cervix**

cervix alters position according to the time of the month and how aroused you are–so don't worry if you 'lose' it occasionally.

If you want you can also buy a speculum, an instrument which allows you to hold your vagina open and explore it more fully. Women's Health (address in the Resource Section) sell a speculum kit that you can use. The speculum is shaped like two shoehorns joined together. When you place it inside the opening to your vagina (warm it first!) the two halves can be eased apart, allowing you to explore your vagina more fully. It

126

is a good idea to use a mirror so that you can see into your vagina, as well as feel inside it.

Whether you are looking or just touching, try to notice as many things as you can. Be aware of moisture or discharge, and of the shape, size and feel of your cervix. Become familiar with these things. Remember that this part of your body is undergoing changes, so it may feel particularly vulnerable at the moment.

The cervix – types of skin

Inside the cervix, beyond the reach of your fingers, the cells of

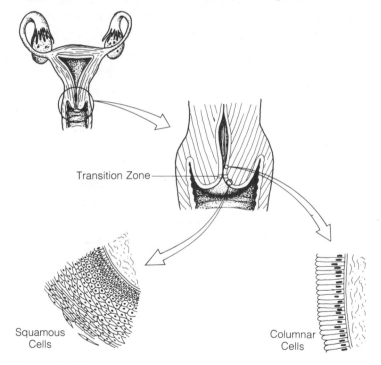

Transition Zone

Squamous Cells

Columnar Cells

Figure 14 **The transformation zone of the cervix**

127

the skin are soft and have a good blood supply. They are called columnar cells. At the outside of the cervix, and in the vagina, the cells are of a different kind: they are called squamous cells and have less of a blood supply than columnar cells, and are 'harder', so that you don't bleed every time you are penetrated when making love.

Between the two types of skin is a transformation zone, where cells change from one kind to another. The soft, columnar cells inside the cervical canal change into harder squamous cells towards the outside of the cervix. This is a way of protecting the vulnerable cervix from the outside world. The medical term for this transition is squamous metaplasia.

You won't be able to feel the different kinds of cell, or feel the change from one kind to another. If you have an internal examination to check your cervix after a positive smear, the consultant may use a high-powered microscope to see the different kinds of cell – and sometimes, if you are interested, s/he can show you photos of your own cervical cells.

What can go wrong

Infections. One thing that can go wrong in your cervix, or vagina, is that you may catch an infection of some sort. Thrush (candida albicans) is a common infection which causes irritation and a discharge. Trichomoniasis and gardnerella both result in a vaginal discharge and possibly pain when you pass water, while chlamydia also gives you irritation around your genitals – although it may produce no symptoms at all. Nowadays all such infections are completely treatable, but they can cause your smear result to be unclear. If you do have an infection, your smear may be difficult to interpret and the doctor will often suggest you have a repeat smear after treatment.

Viruses. Your cervix and vagina may also be attacked by viruses. In particular the viruses that carry herpes and warts. Both viruses are infectious and can be passed on through skin contact.

The herpes virus is caught through skin to skin contact, although some people are immune to it. It can lie dormant, but can also flare up when a person is stressed, to cause red spots which turn to painful, weeping blisters.

Warts are growths that can occur on many parts of the body. They are caused by a virus called human papilloma virus, of which there are several kinds. Certain kinds create genital warts, found on the penis in men and the vagina, cervix and external sexual parts in women. However it often exists in the body without producing warts at all, so it is very difficult to track down. A simple test for penile warts is to swab a mild solution of vinegar and water over the penis – infected areas then show up as small white patches.

Cervical ectropian (erosion). Usually, the cells on the surface of the cervix are hard, squamous cells, and the ones on the inside are the softer, columnar cells. If the softer cells come to the surface of the cervix, this can be a problem. Because they are softer, they are more vulnerable. This is called cervical erosion or ectropian.

It sounds as if the cervix is being rubbed or 'eroded' away, but this is an exaggeration. Cervical ectropian can happen during ovulation, menstruation, in pregnancy, or when a girl starts having her periods, and it can also be caused by the Pill.

Many women get it, and unless you have an abnormal smear, it's usually agreed to be harmless.

Hormonal changes. Different hormonal changes may influence a smear result. Very young women, whose hormones are still settling after puberty; pregnant or post-partum women who are undergoing hormonal changes because of child-bearing; and older women whose hormones are altering because of the menopause, may find that their smear result is unclear or gives a false reading. Often these hormonal shifts look like abnormal cell changes, and a woman who has them may need to go for further examination in order to find out what exactly is happening on her cervix.

Abnormally developing cells. The cells on the cervix can develop in abnormal ways. The cells in the transformation zone are particularly vulnerable to abnormal change and may begin to change towards becoming cancer cells. It is important to realize that this is not a change to cancer, but a change in that direction. It happens gradually and slowly, and there are various stages before the cells become truly cancerous. It can take between ten and twenty years for cells to become cancerous. This is why, of all the cancers we know, cervical cancer is one of the easiest to spot and to stop in good time.

One medical term for such changes in the surface layers of the cervix is dysplasia. Another term is pre-cancer, and this can be misleading, because you can start to think that you are definitely going to develop true cancer. In fact, some abnormally changing cells never develop into cancer, even if they are not treated. A third term to describe abnormal cell changes is cervical intraepithelial neoplasia. If you find this a mouthful, you are not alone! It is such a mouthful that it is usually shortened to CIN. Throughout this book I have preferred to use this expression when discussing early, pre-cancerous changes.

In order to make distinctions between various stages of change, doctors have developed a scale, according to how much of the cervix is affected:

CIN 1 means that only the top third of the cells on the surface of the cervix are affected.

CIN 2 means that two thirds of the cells are affected.

CIN 3 means that all the cells on the surface are affected.

Another way of describing CIN 3 is carcinoma in situ. The word carcinoma means cancer, and if you see this term on your medical sheet, or overhear it, as Anna did ('I heard the consultant say those words on his way into the room to examine me . . .') you may well, as she did, panic. There is no need to. Carcinoma in situ is not yet true cancer, as explained later in this chapter.

To get things in perspective, remember that even if left untreated, many cases of CIN 1 and 2 can go back to normal. It has been estimated that of all CIN 1 cases, 60 per cent will regress, 26 per cent remain exactly the same, and only 14 per cent get worse. Of this last group, it is estimated that only 50 per cent progress to become cancer, and this can take decades to happen. The fact is that most women who have treatment for pre-cancerous conditions never develop full-blown cancer.

Cancer. Beyond the CIN scale are further scales of seriousness. The cells of the cervix may indeed be cancerous.

How does cancer happen? Healthy cells grow regularly by dividing and making more cells. This is how children grow.

131

When this division stops, growth stops – and this is why older people change in their appearance, as cells stop reproducing, and wrinkles begin.

When cells grow at an abnormal rate, and the growth gets out of control, this is called a tumour. It can be harmless (benign) or harmful (malignant). Malignant cells are those which spread far beyond their starting point, and destroy other parts of the body, affecting other areas by creating new tumours called 'secondaries'.

Cervical cancer is almost always caused by abnormal changes in the squamous and columnar cells, as described on page 128. This abnormal change spreads beyond the surface layer of the skin and invades the cervix.

There is another form of cervical cancer called adenocarcinoma[10] which doesn't begin in the transformation zone, but in the tissues of the canal that runs through the cervix. Up to a few years ago, adenocarcinoma seemed extremely rare, though recently, perhaps due to more effective investigation, more cases have been found – up to one in ten of all cervical cancers; the increase seems to be more marked for women under 35. Often, women have both CIN conditions, beginning in the transformation zone, and adenocarcinoma as well. The treatment for adenocarcinoma – cone biopsy or hysterectomy – is the same as that for other cervical cancer.

If left untreated cancer spreads further into the cervix. It can invade the whole of the pelvis, and then attack the lymph nodes and bloodstream.

There are several grades of cancer, just as there are several grades of CIN. Only the very last grades are fatal. The highest mortality rates are found in those women who, unlike you, have never had a smear test.

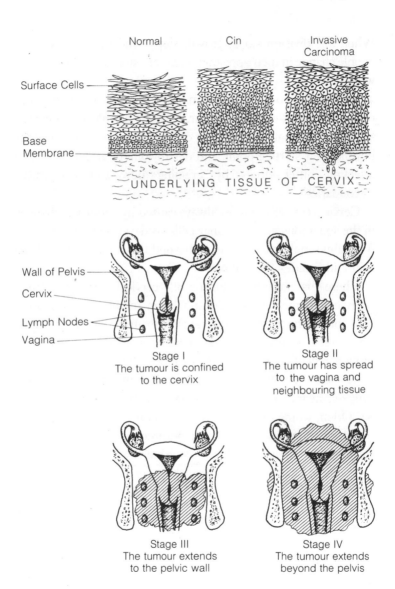

Figure 15 **Stages of CIN**

133

Positive Smear

When is it pre-cancer and when is it cancer?

This is one of the main mixed messages in the whole of the 'positive smear' area. It is confusing because, in the majority of cases, we are dealing with a condition that develops along a continuum. Mild cases are nowhere near being cancerous, more severe cases are more likely to be so.

The dividing line that doctors draw relates to what cancer does: it spreads and grows. This is the very nature of cancer, to grow and invade the body it attacks. So if the condition is not invading the cells at a deep level, it is not regarded as truly cancerous. The words and terminology doctors use refer to whether the condition has started to spread beyond the very surface cells of the cervix. If the condition is only affecting surface cells, it is easily treated and there will be no danger of its having invaded the body. This is the condition that doctors call CIN. It is not seen as cancer yet because it has not yet started to invade. The grades of CIN, as we have seen, refer to the extent to which the cervix is affected by this surface condition – a third (mild), two thirds (moderate) or all (severe). The final grade, CIN 3 is, confusingly, called by the same Latin name as is used for true cancer – *carcinoma* – but if the condition has not yet invaded, it is not seen as true cancer.

If the condition has spread beyond the surface cells of the cervix, then doctors consider it has invaded: they use the term 'invasive carcinoma', and see the condition as cancer. The treatment has to be more searching in order to eradicate all of the affected cells.

A positive smear test only reveals whether the cells are abnormal or not; the term used is whether they are dyskaryotic. If the dyskaryosis is mild, then it is very unlikely

134

that the abnormality has spread so far that it is invasive; if it is moderate or severe, then there is usually little chance. New research has recently revealed that mild dyskariosis with a high level of the wart virus may mean a high grade of CIN, but a smear test alone does not check for CIN or cancer, and you need a biopsy for this.

So if your smear shows mild dyskaryosis, it is practically certain that the condition you have is not invasive and therefore not true cancer. You may have an examination or biopsy to make sure, but minimal treatment will be needed. And as the condition can develop, some doctors will refer you for an examination as a matter of course–particularly as with today's waiting lists, if you need to enter the treatment cycle at all, you need to get in early.

With moderate or severe dyskaryosis, a doctor will usually consider what other symptoms you have if any. S/he will send you to hospital for an examination and a biopsy to make sure that you are not one of the few women who have an invasive condition.

If, when the examinations have been done, you are told you have a CIN condition, you know that the abnormal cells are only on the surface of the skin. Various proportions of your cervix could be affected depending on whether you have CIN 1, 2 or 3, but the condition has not invaded, and is therefore not regarded as cancer. If however it has gone below the surface of the skin, then you are no longer seen as having a CIN condition, but true 'invasive carcinoma'.

The two are on a continuum though, and this is why there may sometimes be confusion. If you have CIN you will be advised to go for treatment because, left alone, it might spread and become invasive cancer–but doctors will still reassure you by saying that it 'isn't yet'. In the same way, advertising campaigns for the smear test talk of cervical cancer, even though the majority of the positive results show CIN conditions, not invasive conditions.

As I mentioned before, the length of time it takes for CIN to turn to cancer, if in fact it does, can be anything up to twenty years–although there seems to be a new, fast developing form of the condition which can become serious in a much shorter time. Doctors are also particularly worried about younger women, whose rates of cervical cancer seem to be increasing very fast.

If you can become clear in your mind about the relationship between the two things, you will be well on your way to avoiding the trap of mixed messages.

What now?

You have now had the benefit of a short guided tour around the facts of a 'positive smear'. It may take some time for you to be able to understand and assimilate these facts. One woman spoke of not being able to 'take anything in until it was all over'. Also, many of these facts are not relevant to you, and you will never need to know them.

Whatever your positive smear means, it is an opportunity to get to know more about your body.

9   What are the causes?

' *I didn't search for reasons or
causes because I wasn't looking for
things to blame.* '

(Julie)

Why is it happening? This is a question that every woman I talked to wondered about. They wondered in a general way and in a specific way, about what caused cervical cancer and CIN. They asked: why is it happening to me?

This question can be a cry to heaven – or whatever your substitute for heaven is. It can be a question that doesn't expect an answer; you simply feel angry and resentful that such a thing can be happening. You have every right to be angry and resentful, for what is happening to you is not pleasant. And if you want to, you can channel your anger into an energy for doing something practical – exploring what laid the foundations for your condition, and what can stop it happening again.

Finding out why

If you do decide to explore these things, you will need all the energy you can get. Because of all the questions surrounding the issue of positive smear, the actual 'cause' of cervical cancer is one of the most difficult.

Doctors disagree, medical professionals argue, the press claims one thing, pressure groups claim another. The women I spoke to came up with several possible links which the professionals had never even considered. If you are looking for clear-cut answers, you won't get them.

You should also be aware that you are touching upon an area in which people may react strongly and negatively. If you decide to explore the issue, you are likely to come across opinions that will upset you, make you angry, put you on the defensive. For people are very ready to blame, dramatize, blandly reassure or simply refuse to comment. As Frances said: 'No one told me why it happened – and I hated that.'

We still don't know for sure what the causes of cervical cancers are: it will take many more years of research, argument and unhappiness before we reach anything approaching a satisfactory answer. All I can offer in this chapter is a path through the minefield, a guide to recent thoughts on the subject.

Causes or promoters?

Let us start by challenging the idea of a 'cause' of cervical cancer and CIN. We are not talking about an injury, such as a broken leg, that is caused by an accident.

We don't yet know what makes a cell decide to grow and go on growing out of control. It is not yet clear what the trigger is. But although we do not know what 'causes' cancer, we do know that certain conditions make the cells more vulnerable to cancer taking hold. So when we talk of causes, we are talking in fact about 'promoters', factors that cause vulnerability.

It is important to remember this. Many newspaper articles, television programmes and top medical consultants forget it. Every factor mentioned here as being present in women who develop cervical CIN or cancer, may also be present in women who don't develop it. So if any of them are present in your life, then that doesn't mean to say you will get cancer. It just means that you are more vulnerable. And the more of these vulnerability-promoters you have in your life, the more vulnerable you are, in the same way as if you go jumping off cliffs you are more likely to get injured than if you stay at home reading. You are not under a death sentence – but you are stacking the odds against yourself.

Promoters

Diet

The links made between diet and cervical pre-cancers and cancers are still uncertain. However, vulnerability is a wide-ranging thing. If your diet is unhealthy or unbalanced; if it gives you fewer nutritional resources to draw on when you are ill; if it makes you severely over or underweight for your size, it's making you vulnerable anyway. Many of the women I spoke to had improved their diet after having a positive smear.

Some foods can lower the efficiency of your immune system which helps you fight disease. Generally, foods which have an adverse effect on any part of your body (such as too much fat, caffeine or alcohol) increase your vulnerability to disease of any kind.

Recent studies on both sides of the Atlantic suggest that women with cervical pre-cancers or cancers often hav⁓ deficiencies of certain elements – vitamin C, bⸯ folic acid. Vitamin C helps to convert harⸯ the blood-stream into non-harmful ones, a uncooked fruit and vegetables. Beta carotene, found in carrots and other yellow vegetables and fruits, helps build up resistance to disease. The contraceptive pill makes it difficult to absorb the folic acid from what you eat, so you are particularly liable to deficiency if you are on the Pill.

Pollution

It has been recognized for a long time that a polluted environment and disease go together. Recent studies[11] have shown a link between 'dirty' jobs and a higher incidence of positive smears in women workers or the wives of male workers. Workers (or their wives) in the forces, the mines, at furnaces and foundries, on farms and on fishing boats, and in mills, have all been found to be more at risk.

Think of the proven risks of asbestos, which now has been removed from work places and schools. It's easy to see why if you work with such high-risk substances you are more vulnerable. If your partner works with them, and you wash her/his clothes, make love with her/him – or even live within breathing distance of the same mill or mine – you are vulnerable too.

It's less easy to see why some people therefore put value

judgments on cervical cancer as an unhygienic disease. It is no more dirty – and no less shocking – than silicosis. It certainly doesn't mean that the sufferer does not wash or care about her personal hygiene. Industrial dirt, diesel fumes and chemicals are not easily washed away; they linger on the skin and in the air. What it means is that some women's vulnerability to such things is in a special, sexual area rather than in a more easily talked about area such as the lungs.

That said, one of the factors which may lead to illness is a lack of good washing facilities. If your work place doesn't have showers, or your house doesn't have a bathroom, you are at a disadvantage. You need to make sure that you get that advantage back, and fight for a better environment. Equally, be aware that some products that may seem to reduce pollution, in fact add to the environmental pressures on your body. Strong douches or vaginal deodorants that destroy your normal vaginal secretions may seem to make you clean, but in fact may be polluting your cervix more than plain water would. Steer clear of douches and perfumed deodorants or wipes.

Lack of knowledge and skill

Why include lack of knowledge and skill as factors that lead to cervical conditions? Vulnerability is not only about being under-nourished or stressed. It is also about being open to attack because you have no defence.

If a woman has no knowledge of what a positive smear means or how to get one, if when she goes to get one she cannot communicate with the doctor, if she hasn't the words or the assertiveness to ask for the treatment she needs, then she is vulnerable. And this can be a factor in the development of CIN, and cancer taking a hold.

There are women without the resources to enter the health service system and fight for what they want[12]. They range from very young women to women who are unable to speak the language of the country they are in, or are unaccustomed to medical practices and bureaucracy. Others may be too old to cope with the red tape and the waiting, or not assertive enough to ask for what they need. All of these women are vulnerable: delays can occur, treatment may be too late or inadequate. The disease develops, not because of what the woman eats, or whether she smokes, but because she cannot get the best from the system.

The problem is not confined to cervical cancer, of course. Women with other medical problems may find themselves in the same situation. Perhaps, though, we need to remember that cervical conditions in particular can make some women embarrassed, and therefore less able to cope.

Lack of medical resources

Doctors themselves can add to a woman's vulnerability by being ignorant or simply not having the time or energy to spare. Some of the women I talked to told me of doctors brushing off their inquiries about smears or follow-up treatment as 'trivial'. It can seem, when your last patient was dying, that the woman who comes with CIN 1 is wasting your time.

All too often, however, doctors are very willing to help, and it is the money and resources that are lacking. Because of lack of government funding, some women may experience difficulty in having smears more than once every few years. Once a smear is taken, the waiting time for diagnosis, and then treatment, can be alarmingly long. The condition can worsen in the interval.

Another 'promoter' of cervical problems, sadly highlighted by several real-life cases over the past few years, is inaccurate results from smear tests, leading to cervical conditions going unsuspected for years. Most smear test laboratories now have quality control systems, but nevertheless, technicians are expected to do many smears a day. More money, time, training and support would help them do their jobs as well as they want to.

Of course, this situation varies depending on the area in which you live. Well-to-do areas often have better screening programmes and bigger hospitals, while poorer areas have long waiting lists and fewer facilities. As always, women who are in lower-paid jobs, unemployed, or at home have less opportunity to change area, or pay for private health care services. This is a promoter of yet another vulnerability.

Tobacco

Most people nowadays know that smoking makes you more vulnerable to lung cancer. What they often don't know is that smoking also greatly increases your risk of getting cervical cancer and CIN. Carcinogens show up in your cervical secretions in ten times the concentration they do in your blood. Smoking twenty cigarettes a day can make you seven times more vulnerable; forty cigarettes a day make you fourteen times more vulnerable.

Smoking is harmful in a number of ways. First, it lowers your resistance to any disease or infection. In a general sense it weakens your heart and lungs, making you more likely to get ill. More specifically, Langerhans cells, which form part of the body's immune system, are reduced by smoking – and studies have shown that these cells are reduced in women with CIN conditions. By smoking, you reduce your body's ability to fight off disease.

Also, the nicotine in cigarettes finds its way into the mucus which covers your cervix. The nicotine actually seeps through into the mucus and affects the cervical cells. Those cells, as we saw in the chapter on Facts, are constantly changing. The presence of nicotine in them destroys the immune system which keeps them healthy, so they are then more likely to change abnormally.

Very few of the women I spoke to smoked. Some of them had, but had stopped after their positive smear. Most of them agreed that smoking made them more vulnerable, although few of them saw a direct link. A few had tried to give up, and couldn't. As Lily said: 'I shouldn't be smoking I know, but at the moment (she was waiting for a further operation) I just can't stop.'

The Pill

When the contraceptive pill first came on the market, it seemed the answer to all our problems. With the arrival of the Pill came the chance for women to choose to have children, responsibly and with awareness. Now it seems that the Pill has a number of side effects. We have all heard horror stories of the Pill, and many of us have suffered our own minor horror stories of weight gain and depression. Although it is still the most reliable form of contraception, it may not, as far as women are concerned, be the 'safest', especially in relation to cervical cancer and CIN.

In the first place, the Pill can reduce our body's natural immunity to infection, making us more likely to fall ill. It can also reduce the body's ability to take in and use folic acid – and recent American work suggests that women with positive smears often have a folic acid deficiency. Next, using the Pill on its own leaves you open to catching a sexually transmitted virus or infection. As later sections of this chapter show, some doctors believe that these viruses are a factor in the development of cervical cancer and CIN. If a woman is not on the Pill, this theory goes, she or her partner usually uses a barrier form of contraception, which protects her. If she is on the Pill, usually they don't, which leaves her more vulnerable.

But does the Pill itself directly create cervical conditions which enable cancer to develop? There is considerable evidence to suggest that women on the Pill develop cervical problems more often than other women do. On the other hand, many doctors say that the Pill is not a factor in cervical cancer. They also point out that the risks to women of not taking the Pill – through abortion and birth complications – can be greater than the risks from taking the Pill. They remind us of studies suggesting that the Pill actually protects us from other forms of cancer, such as ovarian cancer. We are faced with unclear evidence, and this means that it is easy for people to interpret it in whichever way they want.

It is possible that doctors are influenced by the thought of what might happen if all women turned against the Pill. Many women would not want to stop making love spontaneously. And some doctors imagine that, without the Pill, there would be far more unwanted pregnancies. As Sue said: 'They don't want to mention the Pill because it's such a nice, convenient thing.'

This seems to me to be a patronizing attitude to take towards women. Most of us *are* able to think and choose for ourselves, and *can* take responsibility for not 'getting ourselves pregnant'. (The unwritten message in that phrase of course is that women are solely responsible for pregnancy; but it takes two to tango.) In short, if we believe that the Pill makes us vulnerable, we can choose not to take it, and also choose not to get pregnant.

Sexual behaviour

There is much controversy about how (and how far) women's vulnerability to cervical cancer and CIN is linked to heterosexual love-making. Nevertheless, there seems to be considerable evidence to suggest that sexual activity can be one of the promoters of a woman's vulnerability[13]. The main links suggested are these:

> *The earlier a woman first has intercourse, the more vulnerable she is.*

During our teenage years, the soft cells of the vagina and cervix (columnar cells) are replaced by harder (squamous) cells more able to cope with the pressure of penetration. If penetration happens early in our lives, then these cells might not have fully formed. The softer cells can be damaged and made more vulnerable. In addition, intercourse without barrier contraception may make it more likely for a woman to catch a vulnerability-inducing virus or infection.

> *The earlier a woman has her first child the more vulnerable she is.*

This theory is based on the same idea – that early use of the cervix, before the cells are fully formed, may damage it. Also, cervical erosions occur often in women who have had children, and can make women more vulnerable. This idea is mentioned in only some of the literature available, and is not as widely accepted as other theories. However it is also not such good headline material as the next theory:

> *The more male partners a woman has had, the more vulnerable she is. And the more partners her male partners have had, the more vulnerable she is.*

Here again, opinions vary. Many studies claim that women with CIN and cancer often have more than one partner, and these women often have partners who have slept with more than one person. This would suggest that there is some sort of cancer trigger that is being spread to women through men and back again. Some studies suggest that the possibility of cancer is lower when women or their male partners use a barrier form of contraception like the cap or condom, and that using these methods can actually help clear up the condition.

The evidence is not clear cut for any of these sex-link theories, and there is evidence to contradict them or at any rate strongly suggest that other disease promoters may be more important for many women. For example, lesbians who have never made love with a man may still have positive smears, and so may virgins. Many women develop CIN or cancer without having either early intercourse, early childbirth, multiple partners, or any sexually-transmitted problems. However it is certainly true that with condom use, cervical conditions tend to get better of their own accord, which does suggest that some women become more vulnerable to disease when making love with some men.

Adding fuel to the fire, there is still argument about the reasons why the number of sexual partners matters. We still don't know for certain exactly what is the possible 'cancer trigger' that is sexually transmitted. Below are listed some of the theories for what that trigger is. In every case, the research is still ongoing. Also in every case, many women who don't seem to have that particular trigger develop CIN and cancer; and many of us who do carry particular triggers remain healthy and cancer-free.

Possible sexual triggers

Sperm. One theory is that a protein substance in some sperm causes changes in the cells of the cervix. The sperm, thought to be present in certain 'high-risk' men, may be especially dangerous when it touches an unformed, maturing cervix. This fits in with the theory which states that women who make love early are more vulnerable. It also fits with the theory that the more partners a woman takes, the more at risk she is.

Another theory[14] tentatively suggests that substances in the seminal fluid, which carries the sperm and which is necessary to allow fertilization of a woman's egg, may possibly reduce her ability to overcome the disease. If this is so, then whatever risk a woman has of developing cervical cancer may be promoted by unprotected sexual intercourse. This is, obviously, not due to a sexually transmitted disease, but to seminal fluid doing what it is normally and happily meant to do – creating the conditions for conception. Unfortunately, while doing so, it may also create the conditions for vulnerability to any possible disease that might be lurking.

Cancer partners. Partners of men who develop cancer of the genitals often seem to develop CIN and cervical cancer later on. It follows therefore, that the more partners you have, the higher the probability that you will have one partner who later develops cancer and, according to this theory, the greater the risk to yourself. The evidence for this theory is, however, contradictory.

Infections. It has been suggested that sexually transmitted infections can decrease your natural immune system, making you more likely to catch any disease. In particular, they can also increase your vulnerability to cancer. Women with positive smears have been found to have a high incidence of thrush, gardnerella, chlamydia and trichomoniasis.

Infections that cause a discharge may also make it easier for the wart virus to develop in the vagina. The wart virus grows more easily when discharge is present–and as we shall see later, is seen by some to be connected with cancer and CIN.

The herpes virus. Up to a few years ago, the fact that many women with positive smears have the herpes virus was seen to suggest a link between them. Nowadays, the possibility is seen as slim, although further research may re-establish a link. In either case, if you have the herpes virus, you will want it to be treated.

The wart virus. When this book was first published, the wart virus was seen as crucial in the development of abnormal cells. As mentioned in Chapter 8, there are a group of viruses which cause warts in various parts of the body, including the sexual

149

parts. But even when there are no warts to be seen, the wart virus may be present. It will be passed on from partner to partner, and the higher the number of partners, the greater the chance of catching the wart virus.

Some research has suggested that certain varieties of the virus cause changes in cervical cells, making them grow uncontrollably, and that some wart viruses are seen to be responsible for a new, fast-developing form of cancer[15, 16].

Over the last few years, however, many medical professionals have argued against the link[17-20]. They point out that not all women who have CIN or cervical cancer have these wart viruses, so there must be other factors involved. Also, many women who have the wart virus don't develop either warts or CIN. Some estimates say that 70 per cent of the population have the wart virus anyway, so that it would not be surprising that many of the CIN women seemed to have the virus. Finally, there have also been studies which show that, in cases where both the wart virus and CIN are present, even when the wart virus is not cured, most women treated for CIN do not get it again. If a relationship had existed between the two, it could reasonably be supposed that the CIN would have reoccurred. In the face of all this argument and evidence, current guidelines are that women with the wart virus are probably not at increased risk of cervical cancer, and that it is the CIN condition that should alert us to problems, not simply the presence of the wart virus.

Within the past few months, however, new evidence has challenged this. Women with mild dyskariosis who underwent a special test for the presence of the wart virus HPV 16 were found to have a much higher chance of having CIN 3; this strongly suggests a link between the wart virus and CIN conditions. Professionals are beginning to reconsider the evidence.

Faced with such disagreement among the experts, it seems wise for me to continue to include details of the wart virus in this book, and for you to bear in mind that if you know you have the wart virus, treating it will certainly increase your cervical health and may possibly remove yet another promoter of your vulnerability to cancer.

Fact or judgement?

While some studies deny the sexual link with cervical cancer, most support it. But whatever the facts, they are often misinterpreted to include a subtle judgment. Studies often suggest that women with cervical conditions have had a multitude of lovers, and value judgments are being made about that. Unfortunately history adds to the problem. Italian research as early as 1842 concluded that nuns did not get cervical cancer; further research claimed that there was a high frequency of cervical conditions among prostitutes. In much of the literature, therefore, as well as in the media, and from misguided health officials, one finds comments like 'Nuns don't get it . . .' and the concomitant 'Prostitutes do . . .'.

Faced with these claims, we very quickly enter blame territory. This is very disturbing to the many, many women whose sex lives have hitherto been happy and untroubled and who are now suddenly faced with the thought that they, or their partners, have been promiscuous and that this has caused their disease. We can forget that one partner alone can create vulnerability. As one doctor very wisely points out, it is more difficult to treat the marital and sexual problems caused by this blame than it is to treat the cervical cancer itself!

The facts are these. Later studies[21],[22] have totally contradicted the 'nuns and prostitutes' research. They have shown that nuns, as well as virgins, do get cervical cancer, while women with a high rate of sexual partners, such as prostitutes, or women from multiple-partner cultures, can have a lower than normal rate of cervical problems. Also, most women attending colposcopy clinics for treatment have had only one or two partnerships, often in long-term relationships. So as far as the facts are concerned, we are now long past the stage where there is any basis for being judgmental. As far as your personal situation is concerned, this should be true as well. In practice, if you yourself think there is a link between your sexual behaviour and your positive smear, you may want to change what you are doing, maybe using barrier contraception, maybe opting for fewer partners or longer-term ones. But this is your concern alone, a decision you will make in order to lower a risk which is a very real possibility.

In terms of other people's thoughts about your sexual behaviour, however, having a positive smear should never mean that you are judged. In particular, the leap from the statement 'sexual behaviour may be linked with cervical cancer' to 'cervical cancer is something only promiscuous people get' is one which we should all be wary of. For the first statement may be a fact; the second statement can never be anything but a biased value judgment.

Stress

Stress has always been identified as one of the things that stops us being healthy. We get ill more easily, we throw off disease more slowly. Many of the women I spoke to mentioned stress as a factor. They talked of being overworked or worried. And they told me how one of the first things they did after hearing that they had a positive smear was to try to cut down their work load and worry less. 'I've always been a worrier,' said one woman. 'Now I know I must take things easy–I have no choice.'

Past experiences

As I interviewed the women who had contacted me, I noticed a strange pattern emerging. It was not one that has ever been mentioned in relation to positive smears, but it was clearly present. The pattern was this: many of the women I spoke to who had had positive smears had also had in their lives some trauma attached to sexuality or fertility.

Two of the women I spoke to had been raped. Several had had abortions. Many spoke of traumatic relationships: 'It was as if I was being punished for having an abortion'; 'My punishment . . . for the abortion and for people I'd slept with in the past'; 'I always linked my CIN with sleeping with someone when I knew I didn't want to . . .'

I wonder at this. I would not want to suggest that a traumatic incident in early life triggered CIN or cancer or that the stress of early trauma created a vulnerability in which cancer or CIN could develop. And yet the women I spoke to saw a link, even if only in their minds, which caused them pain and guilt. So although doctors and researchers are concentrating on what they think causes cervical disease, I would like to point out that many women make entirely different mental links, which affect the way they think and feel. It would be helpful if doctors were aware of this.

Miscellaneous

Some women I talked to rejected all the theories. Some

153

considered they were just unlucky. Some thought it was just 'one of those things': 'I weighed up all these causes and thought it might not be any of those. So I didn't worry about it too much.' (Rachel).

Others came up with their own, special theories: 'I have a skin condition (psoriasis) in which cells multiply. It seemed as if CIN was the same thing,' said Jane G. 'I'd recently been suppressing a lot of emotion–it was a way of getting rid of all the tension I had down there,' thought Hilda.

None of these things are seriously mentioned in the leaflets or the articles by professionals. Yet they may ring true for you and if they do, perhaps they are more relevant to you than all the research on smoking, and diet and viruses.

Knowing your vulnerabilities

In the end, whatever it is that creates your particular vulnerability is specifically yours. Jane G. said: 'My illness was my illness and to do with me,' and that seems to sum it up. Certainly there is a great deal of evidence which points to links between certain factors and the positive smear. Smoking, the Pill, sexual behaviour all seem to be things to consider carefully.

Considering these factors, you might, perhaps for the first time in your life, have looked at what makes you vulnerable–not only to cervical cancer, but also to a host of other illnesses and diseases. You may now have to rethink your attitude to many things in your life–to partners, to contraception, to yourself.

You may, on consideration, decide to change nothing. But now at least you have some idea of the odds.

❸   **the feelings**

10   Feeling good about yourself

*' I was dealing with it very well
. . . it was me, and I was dealing
with it . . . '*
(Julie)

Some illnesses come and go and leave you as you were before. You still have no less, or no more liking for yourself than you ever had. You don't (usually) cut your arm and spend time feeling guilty that you were clumsy enough to do so.

Having a positive smear can be very different. I did speak to women who saw it as just another illness. But for surprisingly many, it was 'not the same as a cut on your arm'. As Vivienne commented, 'To say that I was difficult to live with is an understatement. I would go from the darkest moods to an unnatural high, from laughter to tears. I was just plain scared.' There are hidden and not-so-hidden messages surrounding the condition, hinting that maybe this time it is your fault, or causing you to think that you shouldn't feel quite so good about yourself as you did before, or that women in general are to blame.

157

If we are to recover fully from a cervical condition, and if we are, socially, to avoid victim-blame, then we need to look at these messages carefully and work out ways to deal with them.

Messages from the past

Where do we get the messages about our own worth? The foundations are laid early on in life: some of these messages may lie dormant for years, then suddenly reappear, precipitated by an event in your life. So if at some time in the past, you got the message that making love was wrong, if when you were small you were told that a doctor was a god-like creature – then these messages may still be with you. They are probably all the stronger because they've been with you for longer. You may believe them without question.

Then they are reactivated by cues from your present situation. If, like Emma, you get a doctor who 'made me feel in the way', then the chances are that this will increase any emotional vulnerability you already have, making you feel even more vulnerable.

Many of the women I spoke to admitted that before the smear, they had had negative feelings about themselves – their health, their sexuality, their emotions. The experience of the positive smear set everything off again. As Judith said: 'I was raped when I was sixteen and the positive smear brought it all back; I had to go through it all again.' This is a very dramatic example. But even a slight lack of self-esteem, common to most women in our society, can be intensified by the news of a positive smear.

The cues

What are the cues that trigger negative feelings? They can be very personal ones; your partner's reaction, for example: 'There's nothing the matter with you – what are you going on about . . .' Many women found that if people who were close thought worse of them for having a positive smear, they began to think worse of themselves.

But the cues can come from much less intimate sources. If a doctor speaks to you in a patronizing manner; if a consultant says that the fact that you sleep with your boyfriend could have created your problem, it can be enough to set you off on a spiral of self-blame. It's important to realize that often, when women are dealing with medical professionals, they start by believing that 'the doctor is always right.' And if s/he is right about the disease and the treatment, then s/he must be right in his/her judgement of you.

Finally, you can be affected by 'what the papers say'. The press, television and radio are often very supportive of the cervical cancer cause. However sometimes they simply get it wrong, as an unfortunate article in a leading women's magazine recently did when it identified women at risk from cervical cancer as being 'promiscuous smokers, basically'. And sometimes the press are also tempted by a good headline to create stories that make the truth unhelpful: 'Two thousand women a year die of guilt . . .' shrieked a tabloid story that linked the (true) fact that some women are wary of going for a smear lest they be stigmatized, and the (true) fact that two thousand women a year die of cervical cancer, to come up with a headline that may have sold papers but did nothing to encourage a change in social attitude. Is it any wonder that we feel bad when faced with publicity like this?

Many of the women I spoke to admitted feeling bad about themselves at some time after hearing the positive smear news. Sometimes this self-doubt lasted minutes, in some cases months. Frances said that she still, a year later, didn't feel as confident as she used to before it happened.

Self-blame

And what are the things that we worry about – what particular issues carry all these feelings of self-blame? There seemed to be a number of them; here is how women expressed them:

'I'm not healthy'

Some women felt bad about getting ill in the first place. Particularly if they'd been very healthy before, they thought that somehow their bodies had let them down. Rachel's very perceptive consultant commented that: 'many women who thought they were healthy get their self-esteem knocked when it happens.'

Once 'it' has happened, if you don't get better on your own, you can feel even worse. Several of my interviewees, particularly those who believed in the power of the mind over the body, were concerned if their efforts at self-cure failed. Julia was 'a bit disappointed as I'd hoped I could make it go away.'

It is certainly true that having a positive smear reminds

many of us of our mortality. It is even more striking because in most cases there are no symptoms, no visible signs, to tell us that something is wrong. And as one woman put it: 'I realize that I can never be totally certain of my health again.'

It may also mean that we simply adapt to this new awareness of our vulnerability. Now that we are aware of it, and can take steps, the vulnerability itself can actually be neutralized. Before, when we were unaware, we were doing nothing about it. Now at least we can take action.

'I'm dirty'

As we explained in the chapter on Causes, poor living and working conditions can make you more vulnerable to cervical disease. Industrial dirt, diesel fumes and lack of washing facilities can create just the right conditions for its development.

For some reason, this fact often gets interpreted as meaning that cervical cancer is a disease of women who are 'dirty', and lots of women take this message on board. Julie 'imagined this tacky, dirty, ugly, black-looking cervix . . .' and not surprisingly felt bad about it.

For this reason cervicography, where you get to look at and often take away with you a photograph of your cervix, may be reassuring. You will be able to see the sheer normality of your vagina. In fact, cervical cancer as a dirty disease is one myth we can dispel at once. It is not a disease of unhygenic women. It is a disease of an unhygenic environment.

'It's my fault'

This was a common reaction. Women convinced themselves that

161

there must be a chain of cause and effect and that they were therefore the cause. Surely, this thinking went, if we have this condition, it must be due to something that we have done.

Two women spoke about their abortions, and made an emotional link between the self-blame they were feeling now and the guilt they felt when they had the abortion: 'I've really regretted that, and the threat of a cone biopsy, which at the time I thought might affect my ability to have children, seemed the worst thing that could happen to me,' said one.

Many women mentioned feeling uneasy about sex. There is a creeping fear that if you hadn't slept with him, then you might never have got . . . that infection, that virus, that CIN, that cancer. So of course it is *your* fault.

In practical terms, remember that talking about fault is inaccurate. The fact that you have a cervical condition is not anyone's fault. Even if there is a connection between sex and cervical cancer, you did not create it. You merely caught it from someone else, who caught it from someone else. You are a victim, not someone to be blamed. Remember too that your cervical condition may well have been caused by one of the many other contributing factors. No one can ever tell you that it is your sex life that is to blame – or that it is your fault.

Often though, the guilty emotion isn't even based on the knowledge that there may be a direct link between penetrative sex and cervical cancer. For there is still a feeling abroad that it is bad to have intercourse, that in some way, if anything bad happens that has a sexual link, then we are getting our just deserts.

You may or may not regret having slept with male partners. If you do regret any of these partnerships, then that is most likely due to the relationship you had with that person. For a doctor, or anyone else, to ask you to start regretting a previously regret-free relationship because now, months or years later, you have an illness of a sexual part of your body, is unacceptable. Don't give in to it.

'People will think I'm promiscuous'

This self-doubt is not an idle fear. Whilst publicizing the first edition of this book, I ended up in a taxi driven by a man who, on hearing what my book was about, grunted 'Wouldn't give these women house room ... it's all caused by sleeping around.' When faced with the reality of a positive smear, then, women like Linda worry that 'people will point a finger at me ...' and some women were actually confronted by friends and relatives: 'My husband's mother rang me one evening to say that she'd heard you only get it if you're promiscuous. I said to her – I've only slept with one man and that's your son,' reported one woman.

If you are heterosexually active, you may have had one male sexual partner, or several. That is a fact and is indisputable. A negative comment on that fact may be someone else's view, but it does not have to be yours. Sleeping with X number of partners is a fact. To define this as 'promiscuous' is a value judgment, and demeaning to you and your relationships. If you are happy with the number of people you have slept with, then no one else has the right to comment, let alone criticize.

So don't fall for it when you read the newspapers, or switch on the television. Don't fall for it when colleagues joke, or friends insinuate. Above all, don't fall for it if partners blame. If you don't fall for it, agree with it, or collude with it, then gradually people will learn that it is not to be done. Facts are one thing, value judgments are another.

'This issue is at odds with my sexuality'

Cervical conditions are seen, all too often, by professionals and lay people, as a disease of actively heterosexual women, but this is not the case. Lesbian women and celibate women do get positive smears, and the problems for them may be made much worse by the fact that they will be treated as if they are actively heterosexual. If you are lesbian or celibate, you may be faced with questions that are embarrassing, examinations that are distressing, and a constant pressure to present yourself as other than you are – and all this may eat away at your self-esteem. In a world that all too often defines women by their ability to relate to men, it is difficult to be completely unaffected by such suppositions. The key, said Amy, is to 'get support from those who know, love and understand you. Then, if you are able to, make the point openly to professionals that women with positive smears are not necessarily all active heterosexuals!'

'I might not be able to have children'

Some women I spoke to, particularly if they were young and had not yet started a family, felt bad because they were afraid their ability to have children had been affected. You can feel very down if that aspect of your womanhood is important to you and is under threat – and your negative feelings could well rebound on you.

If you have had a hysterectomy, then obviously childbearing is impossible. And if this is so, you may feel understandably depressed. Hysterectomy support groups could help you recover your self-esteem and work through your sense of loss.

If you have not had a hysterectomy, it is unlikely that your child-bearing ability will be affected. Occasionally a cone biopsy may make having children more tricky, which is why it is more often used for older women who have completed their families. If you are worried about this and have been advised to have a cone biopsy, then check with your doctor whether you really do need one.

Treatments such as loop diathermy or laser will almost certainly have no adverse effect on your ability to bear children. On the contrary, the removal of abnormal cells and the consequent improvement of your general health, will probably have also improved your chances of having a healthy family.

'I might die'

As mentioned before, death from cervical conditions is extremely rare. But this doesn't mean to say that no woman is ever afraid. If you do feel frightened, then you are not alone; a large proportion of women, even with CIN conditions, were afraid at some point during the process.

The thing to do is to accept that you have a right to be frightened and that being so doesn't mean you are weak. Then remember that there is in all probability no reason for you to be so frightened; the overwhelming majority of women with a positive smear do not have cancer, and the overwhelming majority of those with cancer have never had a smear test at all, so you are, by virtue of having had a test, on the winning side. If you are worried, check with your doctor about the seriousness of your condition; tell him you would prefer to know the truth and cope with it than be denied the possibility of coping by not knowing.

'I feel dependent on the doctors'

A lot of women's lack of confidence sprang from their relationship with the doctors dealing with their case. We'll be looking more closely at the relationship between patients and doctors in Chapter 13. For now, let's look briefly at what can happen with medical professionals that reduces a woman's self esteem.

A woman can feel dependent on the professionals, doctors and nurses, and often the way procedures are set up encourages this feeling. Having to undress and then lie in a vulnerable position to be examined also makes us feel powerless.

The attitude of doctors can make things worse. I know that many doctors are caring human beings who respect and admire the women they treat. But far too many of my interviewees had come into contact with doctors who were not like this. There were many reports of questions going unanswered, and also many complaints about doctors being patronizing or 'talking down' to their patients. When women tried to discuss treatment, they were often met with an unwillingness to accept the possibility that they have any say in the matter.

Happily, many of my interviewees came to their own decisions and voted with their feet. Some changed doctors, others fought for, and got, the treatment they wanted. So they were able to overcome their feelings of dependence and powerlessness. They replaced them, not with feelings of power over the doctors, but with a feeling of being respected and involved in the process of their own health.

'Maybe the treatment will hurt'

Of course you are scared that your treatment, whatever it is, will cause you pain. If you are having a hysterectomy, or any of the radical treatments, then the chances are that you probably will suffer, pain, exhaustion and depression. The answer is to get as much support as you can, physical and emotional.

If you are having one of the treatments for CIN, you may be tempted to feel that you shouldn't be scared. In fact, most women are. And whilst local anaesthetic and sympathetic staff will take most of the discomfort away before it even starts, you may still feel nervous beforehand. Again, however 'mild' your condition and your treatment, get all the support you need and want; you deserve it.

'Maybe I shouldn't be making all this fuss'

Many women cope beautifully with having a positive smear, whether that means cancer or CIN. But we don't all respond

167

like this. Many of us panic even before we know we have a serious illness, and get very emotional if we find out we have. In particular, I found many women with CIN who had been frightened, angry, guilty and sad while at the same time knowing that their condition was not serious and that they would soon be well.

Sometimes feeling all these emotions can seem self-indulgent: 'You feel wicked, going on about it for so long . . .' said Anna, who had a CIN condition. Three months after her operation, she burst into tears when her GP asked her how she was. The doctor, understanding what was happening to her, listened for a while and then put her in touch with a counselling service.

Sometimes the response is not quite so positive. Linda's husband commented: 'What's all the fuss about – you haven't got cancer,' and this can be the attitude of many partners, friends and doctors. There is a mixed message here: while on the one hand you need to take the condition seriously, have regular smears, and take precautions against it deteriorating, on the other you have to bear in mind that your condition is nevertheless minor, though it might not seem minor to you.

If you have to have more aggressive treatment, you can still feel just as confused – and could get the same response from people who are trying to help. 'They kept saying "It's nothing" but it wasn't nothing to me,' said Diana about her hysterectomy. If you know that you have a serious disease, you need two things: firstly some hope that it is going to be all right, and secondly the opportunity to cry and scream and shout if you feel like it, because all this is happening to you.

Guilt about these feelings can be eased. You can ask people not to tell you that 'it's nothing'. You can ask them to support you whether or not they feel that your fears are groundless. You can also remember that one of the reasons they want to reassure you is that your fears and your anger make them feel bad; they are simply protecting themselves against their own emotions by asking you to dampen down yours.

Feeling good about yourself

Lots of women coped with their positive smear experience and gained extra strength from it. They were able to look back afterwards and feel good about what they had done.

Sue said that after her hysterectomy, she often reminded herself what she had to be glad of in her life: 'With a little formula . . . I'm still alive, I don't have periods anymore . . .' She, and many of the other women, talked about 'coming through it all', and how they felt that it was something to be proud of. They felt relief, gratitude, euphoria and an energy to get on with life that simply hadn't been there before.

Perhaps you think that being asked to find positive things in an illness is rather too much of a challenge for many women. If so, all I can say is that in that case many of us have a remarkable capacity for rising to the challenge.

Many women used the experience to get more in touch with what they needed. Being ill and feeling vulnerable seemed to help them to realize that they had to take better care of themselves. Many improved their diet, or their exercise habits. Many gave up smoking. One woman began taking holidays for the first time, and almost all said that they had recognized a need to relax and lead a less stressful life. Some reported changing to forms of contraception they felt were more healthy.

In the same way, having a positive smear helped women to get in touch with what they wanted. Many women had to do this in order to survive. They fought hard to get the doctors they wanted or the treatment they wanted. One woman refused to agree to a hysterectomy until after an exploratory operation. Another went on an assertiveness course to help her cope. Many of the women who went through the positive smear experience learned, as Jane G. did, that: 'We can find out what it is we need, and we can make a choice and get it.'

Many women came through the experience not only with more strength for themselves, but also with more strength for others. When it is all over, and you begin to have time for other people again, then the very fact that you have been through it could mean that you want to help other women. This is a way of feeling good about yourself, too.

'I can help other people because I was helped. I feel good about that,' says Diana, who now writes positive smear advice leaflets for her local gynaecological clinic. It is good to add that, the years since this book was first published, many of the women involved have continued to grow, develop, help themselves and help others. The Positive Smear Conference Update Report showed 'a real upsurge in confidence . . . assertiveness . . . hope'. Lily Hopkins, who at the time the book was written had just gone on television to plead the cause of women in her area whose smear results had been wrongly diagnosed, has now set up self-help groups, a help line and a lecture service. She says ' ". . it has grown into a mini-organization, and as one doctor remarked, "you have a job for life". He is right. I am just as committed today as I was when I first began.'

11 Building your own support system

' My sister was invaluable...
she just wouldn't let me give up '
(Heather)

You may think of yourself as already being part of a wide social network. You may be a loner, and getting support is not something you find easy. But you will handle the positive smear experience better if you find out just what sort of support system you need, and then get it for yourself.

What sort of support system do you need?

A support system can be many things. Some women mentioned wanting sources of information, to help them in their discussions with doctors. And if this is true for you, then good links with local libraries, or the district women's centre or health centre will be all you need. You might need the support of another person here too: Heather's sister 'marched me round to all the libraries to follow up references.'

You may need very practical help, such as child care while you attend appointments or someone to buy your food while you are convalescing after a cone biopsy. It is a good idea to sit down at each stage in the experience, and work out exactly what you need and how to get it. One woman arranged a rota of friends to take her for radiotherapy; they took turns to collect her and bring her back, and then settled her in bed for a rest and a hot drink.

For most of us, support also means being able to talk about what is happening. You might need an occasional chat, in order just to begin to assimilate the experience. You might on occasions need someone with you for a longer period of time, to allow you to feel safe and cared for. On my return from my operation, a friend stayed with me overnight – not so much because of my physical condition, but because I just felt weepy.

It is worth asking yourself what you particularly need from people in the way of emotional support, for we are all different: Julie 'needed to feel I was coping on my own'. Judith 'told everyone'. Some women feel the need to be allowed to cry and get angry when they want to. Others like to feel that they are coping by forgetting that it is happening and doing things that take their mind off the problem. So stop and think just what your needs are, at various times, and with various people: to be held, talked to, allowed to talk, supported in feeling your emotions, distracted from the problems, told 'it's OK', told 'it's OK to be frightened.'

Who can support you?

The support system that you want might not be full of people.

You might prefer to cope on your own. But if you do need people support, whom do you need? You may get help from parents, from children, from family, from friends, from colleagues – and from professional helpers of all kinds. I have not included here the particular support you can get from your intimate partner, because getting support from a partner can often raise problems – and opportunities – that just don't occur in other situations. Chapter 12 covers this in more detail.

Family support can often be the strongest and most binding kind. When you have known someone from birth, you are likely to want to fight to keep them healthy and happy. Viki and Anna, mother and daughter, both had CIN conditions within a very short time of each other: 'Anna was with me through the whole thing and she was very helpful,' said Viki. Heather's sister commented: 'I was determined to support her well.'

Friends, on the other hand, can give much more objective support. They can tell you, where perhaps your mother wouldn't, when you are panicking too much and when you are not standing up for yourself. One friend I had came round when I heard the news, armed with a bottle of wine and a calm: 'Now, I've just seen a television programme, and it said that what you've got is totally curable. So stop whingeing.'

Colleagues are perhaps the least concerned; they may not know you well, or be able to appreciate your emotions. Also, mixing emotions or illnesses with the work situation may be frowned upon. Few of the women I talked to felt able to confide in colleagues or use them as part of an ongoing support system, although one woman told a story of a delightful female boss who allowed her limitless time off for hospital appointments.

173

It is possibly most difficult to know how to relate to children.
They do give support, by being there and by giving affection.
But it's difficult to tell them what is going on – and they could
be upset that Mummy seems absent-minded all of a sudden,
or keeps having to go off and leave them with friends. Few of
the women I talked to had told their children what was
happening because their families were too young. Only Jane B.
had told her teenage daughter that she was starting a cancer
support group, and received the ultimate accolade: 'I think you
could do it, Mum!'

Let's look then at some of the things that might stop the
people around you from giving you really good support.

Blocks to support

Embarrassment

Firstly, you may find it quite difficult to confide, particularly in
older members of your family, about what is happening to you.
Your mother, father and older relatives may be so different
from you in their attitudes, beliefs and ways of helping that
you'd really rather not say anything to them. 'I couldn't tell my
parents,' said more than one woman.

Why can't you confide in other people? Very often it is
because of the stigma attached to a sexually-linked disease.
More than one woman had heard her parents repeat stories
about 'promiscuity and the smear test'. Anna recounts: 'I
didn't tell my colleagues because I'd heard various derogatory

comments about women with positive smears.' Knowing that it might not be easy to explain all the mixed messages that exist around the issue, you may choose not to tell anyone, particularly if your condition is not serious.

If you do tell people, then be prepared for a variety of responses. You may have to face talk about promiscuity or challenges to your sexual life. If you can, explain to people who give you this sort of reaction that the hype about multiple sexual partners just isn't true. Even sleeping with one man – which is something every Mum has done – will put you at risk. Janet reported that her mother, who was very supportive in many ways, commented: ' "I've never had it. Why have you got it?" I thought – it's because you're lucky, Mum.'

Fear

Equally, both relatives and friends will often find it difficult to cope with the possibility of your being seriously ill; they may panic unnecessarily. If it is clear that you have cancer, they might be so distressed at the thought of losing you that they prefer not to talk about it: 'I couldn't talk to my family because they didn't want to be reminded of it,' says Sue.

Even if it isn't clear, they may be so paralysed by the thought that they find it hard to handle: 'I knew your parents had both died of cancer recently,' said one of my close friends, 'so when you had a positive smear, I just thought: "Oh, God, it's happened again", and the thought was very hard to handle.'

Lack of understanding

A final block to getting the support you really want may be that you feel unable to talk to someone who hasn't already had the condition. You imagine that they can't begin to understand what it is like. In some cases your imagination is correct – people who haven't been through it might not be able to realize what you are feeling: 'I don't know anyone in my circle of friends who has it . . . I haven't told them,' said Frances.

On the other hand, many other people have been ill, have felt frightened, have suffered in similar ways to you – even if they haven't had a cervical condition. So don't draw back from asking simply because you are, as one woman put it, 'afraid their guts may turn'.

Helping and being helped

In fact, for many women support meant talking to others in the same situation. And this is a very real option in building your support system. Contacting other women who have had positive smears has two advantages. It means that you are always talking to someone who understands, and it means you are helping while at the same time being helped.

It also means that women are helping themselves and each other; this process can have amazing results. Lily's support group, set up after a misdiagnosis of smear tests in Liverpool, went on to gain national TV coverage and compensatory legal action. So it seems relevant to deal at length in this chapter with how to set up women's networks which can support us in a very special way.

Networking

Many of the women I spoke to had used their experience to communicate and exchange ideas with others. Some of them had used support groups mentioned in the Resource section – The Hysterectomy Support Group and various cancer support groups seemed particularly helpful. It seems, though, that there are very few groups specifically for women who have just had a positive smear. In response to this, four of the women I interviewed had set up support groups and telephone networks to provide on the spot help and support when it is most needed. Their groups met regularly; their telephone network operated when and where it was needed.

It should be remembered, however, that different women have different needs from such a network, in that their illnesses differ. One woman may need counselling after she has heard she has cancer; another may be deeply distressed at having CIN 1. The problems of someone struggling to accept that she has the wart virus and a CIN condition may be very different from those of a woman who has just completed radiotherapy.

The first thing to remember is that in some ways, the more you can specify who you are networking with, the better it will be. A network for women with cervical cancer, a network for women after hysterectomies, a network for women with CIN – all of these will bring together women with the same sorts of problem and in need of the same sorts of help. You may find, of course, that the number of women who respond in your area is so small that you need to widen your scope to include all types of cervical problem. One successful group opens its doors to healthy women too, to learn about their bodies and gain and give support for gynaecological health.

177

Positive Smear

A second thing to remember is that most positive smear women will have their condition for no more than a year, and probably a lot less. So you need to build into your networking some sort of consistency, if there is not to be such a through-flow of members that everyone feels uncomfortable. Find one person, someone who has had a positive smear, but who can keep the energy going to continue organization even when her own condition has cleared up; she needs to be a constant factor, a sheet anchor to give women a sense of familiarity and therefore confidence. If, incidentally, you are thinking of starting a network that includes cancer sufferers, you may need specialized help. The organization Cancerlink provides a service for people who are founding local self-help networking; it offers support, information and training to get you started and help you carry on.

Running a telephone network

In order to set up a telephone network, you will probably need a central organizer who will take the names and numbers of women who are interested in talking to other women. The most active organizational system I found was that at Women's Health, a London-based information centre for women. When women ring with cervical problems, they are asked if they would be willing to talk to others in the same position. If so, their names, addresses, telephone numbers and a short description of their condition is noted down. If necessary, and if the woman prefers, just a first name and phone number can be taken. They are then asked if they would like to talk to someone, and if so, their situation is matched with that of another woman on the network, and the two are put in touch with each other. Being on the network doesn't mean that you spend vast amounts of time helping others – in the four years I've been involved, I've been rung perhaps ten times. But it does mean that a woman who needs to talk has immediate access to someone who can give them a little support, confidentially and often even anonymously.

Running a support group

A support group needs a lot more resources to set up. You need a meeting place and a date that is regular enough for women to know when to turn up. You usually need someone to facilitate the discussion each time, otherwise participants can feel that their needs are not being met. Many groups arrange for a different woman to take on this role each time, and invite guest speakers such as doctors or pathologists to give their viewpoint.

Women who have had a positive smear may need a good deal of information, particularly on the distinctions between cancer and pre-cancer, and the issues around what has caused their condition. Be careful, though, of falling into the trap of 'bowing to the experts', inviting professionals along for the sake of it. Remember too that the main aim of support groups is support; although some women need information, some actually find too many facts disturbing and many do not need information nearly so much as they need to know that they are still valid human beings.

Remember that support groups are a real chance for women to start believing that their experiences are important. It is crucial to allocate a considerable part of each meeting to 'going round the circle', letting each woman give an account of where she is in the process, what has been happening to her since the last meeting, and what her needs are at present. You will find that you don't need to 'set a topic' – the women themselves will talk about what they need to talk about. All the group needs to do is to make sure no one hogs the limelight, and that no one criticizes anyone else for what they say. Ideally, this should be a time for being able to talk freely and openly without fear of rejection, and you should ask all the women in the group to promise to keep the confidentiality of anything that is said 'within these four walls', otherwise people may not feel safe to talk about what is really important to them.

There is a fear, both for women in support groups and those who think of telephone counselling, that somebody you are with will break down completely and you won't be able to handle it. This can happen, but it rarely does, for one very good reason. Human beings are good at self-preservation, and if you feel uneasy – or the support group doesn't feel safe – then women won't let go of their emotions completely. They just won't want to do it. Also, my own experience is that if a woman does feel safe enough to cry, or to talk about her experiences in a very deep way, then the whole group feels better. Each woman can learn something from that.

The book *In Our Own Hands*, by Shiela Ernst and Lucy Goodison (The Women's Press, 1982), has some excellent information about setting up groups of all kinds. Some of the suggestions for games or 'ice-breakers' can be very valuable, particularly if a group knows each other well.

Remember that, as I mentioned earlier, support groups can suffer from rapidly changing clientele. If a group meets once a month, then allowing for holidays and absences, each woman will attend on average a maximum of seven times – one study of a group in London estimated an average of three times only. So it is a good idea to have an anchor person, at whose house the group regularly meets, and who is always there as a familiar face.

Publicizing networks

No telephone or group network will get off the ground unless people know about it. If you do decide to start one, then here are some helpful hints.

Contact your Community Health Council for the names of women's groups and health centres. Try also to find out the names of GPs in your area. Then prepare a simple poster giving the name of the network, a few words about what it does, a contact name and number. If you can, get copies put up in doctors' surgeries, health centres, and anywhere where women with positive smears may go, and you will find the word spreading. Add to this publicity by placing free ads in local news-sheets, district magazines, women's centre papers.

If you want to go more public, then contact your local newspaper and radio station. They are often glad to include a mention of your project on an afternoon programme aimed at women. Suggest to them that they interview someone (perhaps you) involved in the network who can give an idea of what it does and who it is aimed at.

Tell an anecdote or two to convince women that they are not alone in how they feel. And make sure you include your telephone number. If the interview is recorded, stand by your

181

phone afterwards. If it is live, then either get another member of the network to be by the phone – or rush home as soon as you can. 'I got twenty-five phone calls the evening after my interview,' said Lily, 'and the phone didn't stop ringing for days.'

Winding up a support system

Since this book was originally written, many networks for women with positive smears have folded, and new ones have been set up. The Update Report of the Positive Smear Conference highlighted the fact that though there are now more support groups than there were, they tended to have a short lifespan. At first, this worried me, but on reflection, perhaps it is to be expected. Once your condition is cleared, you rarely need support long-term, even though at the time, networking may have been your lifeline to survival.

Perhaps we need to accept that networks, particularly those set up for women with CIN conditions, come and go. This not only means that if you initiate a network, it may well naturally fold; it also means that there is a continuous need for such networks, just as there is a continuous stream of women having positive smears. If your network, telephone service or group seems to be dwindling, first make a concerted effort on the publicity. Perhaps initially, people knew about you; now, posters are old and have been taken down, while the radio interview you gave has been forgotten. So contact doctors, clinics and hospitals again, seek more media publicity, and keep doing it. Only stop if you are convinced that, in your area at least, the need has subsided.

If you do decide that your network is not viable any more, turn your attention to any women who are still in need, waiting for treatment or working through the emotional after-effects. Perhaps arrange a meeting, or ring round to tell them what is happening. Which of them still need support? If a group is not viable, perhaps you can pair them off to support each other? Alternatively, contact one of the existing, and probably more long-lasting cancer support groups in your area, and see if they can offer help. Make sure that not only does each member know there is still support available should they need it, but that they also know that you do not feel disappointed because they do not need you any more. Remember that networks rarely fold because of bad management; rather, they fold because they have done their job and people within them have moved on. There is no need to feel a failure – it may be a sign of success that your work is no longer necessary!

Support systems – the professionals

At the time this book was first written, it seemed as if 'the system' offered little to support positive smear women. Individual professionals were deeply committed to supporting their individual patients, but in general a lack of time and money, and a belief that there was little distress surrounding the issue of a positive smear, meant that few clinics were able to offer real help. I commented, in 1989, that the medical profession often 'didn't seem to know the need existed'.

I am delighted to say that this attitude has shifted considerably. Most professionals now accept the need for counselling, seeing it as a real way not only to ease the trauma of a positive smear for women, but actually to aid healing, reduce recovery time and boost health. All over the country, clinics are attempting to build into their service counselling for colposcopy and treatment. Nurses are pressing for counselling training, and patients themselves are demanding emotional support. The time and the money, however, are still hard to come by: for every clinic which has introduced counselling, there are perhaps another dozen which would like to but are hamstrung by their budgets.

If you are one of the lucky women who is offered counselling at her appointment, and you feel any need of it whatsoever, then grab it with both hands. You will not only be doing yourself a favour, you will be hastening your recovery and also proving to the system that there is a need. If you do not get offered counselling, shout about that as loud as you can.

Counselling in a professional context may, however, be a very different experience from that of offering and being offered untrained support in a network or support group. Firstly, counselling is one-way. You don't need to give anything back, as you might feel you have to when talking to a friend. This is your time, to talk about your concerns, to express your emotions, to confide your worries. A counsellor will keep what you say to her totally confidential, and she will be experienced in dealing with even the strongest emotions, such as anger, fear and grief. She will be well able to help you look back over your life to times when traumatic events happened, and to look forward to changing your life if that is what you want to do. She will not (or should not) offer you advice, but will simply ask questions that allow you to explore your thoughts and feelings.

There are only a few things to be wary of in counselling. Firstly don't feel that it is expected of you to scream and shout. You can do, but simply talking to your counsellor will help if that is what you feel like doing. Secondly, if you do find that you are beginning to explore huge issues in your session – such as the fact that you are having doubts about your partnership, or that you were once raped – then be sure to arrange for further counselling. Once you have dipped a toe in the water of these issues, they will bubble up again in your thoughts, and the one or two hours offered as part of positive smear support will not be enough to deal with them.

Your counsellor, employed only to work in the clinic, may well refer you to another organization, or counsellor, if you wish to carry on exploring your feelings. Alternatively, you can yourself go to one of the counselling organizations mentioned in the Resource section, or find a professional counsellor to work with you. Many of these services cost money; some are free or ask only for a donation. If you need further information to help you find a counsellor, and begin counselling, *The Best Counselling Guide* (Thorson's, 1991) may be of use to you.

Whether you choose to cope with your distress alone, find friends, go to a professional or join a network is up to you. The important thing is to realize that we as women can help ourselves to feel better about things. And, particularly if women help each other, having a positive smear can teach us that we can both give, and ask for, support – perhaps for the first time in our lives.

185

12 Intimate relationships

' I'm Emma's best friend . . . if I
hadn't have been, it would have
all been so much easier. '
(Alain, Emma's husband)

Of all the areas of importance that women talked about to me through many interviews, one of the key ones was that of intimate relationships. 'When you touch your cervix, you touch your heart,' as Jacqui said.

So this chapter looks at all aspects of the intimate relationship as it is affected by the positive smear experience. How do we feel about our partners after a positive smear? What do partners really feel when we are going through our experience of the condition? How can we work together to make the experience a positive one for the relationship?

Setting the framework

But what is your intimate relationship? For the purposes of this chapter, I am assuming that it involves sex. I know that many people who regard themselves as having an intimate relationship, many people who see themselves as partners, don't sleep together. Where cervical conditions are concerned, however, I found that there were particular issues, and particular challenges, to be found within relationships that involved sex.

The main focus of these rewards and challenges is bound to be the relationship or relationships you are in at the time you experience the positive smear process. Most of the women I talked to had one central relationship at that time, although a few women had more than one. And this in itself can cause problems: 'I didn't want my husband to be there when I was treated, I wanted my lover to be there,' said Evelyn. But for the general purposes of this chapter, I shall speak as if you have one current relationship.

Equally, I shall also, in the main, be talking about heterosexual partnerships. Lesbian women do get positive smears, and that means that they and their lovers are deeply affected; I hope that I am, throughout this chapter as throughout this book, aware of the particular suffering that positive smears bring to lesbian women. But when I was talking to women about their feelings, whatever their current sexual status, it was more often than not the heterosexual partnerships, past or present, that triggered their distress and created their negative feelings. Therefore the main direction of this chapter is devoted to that topic.

The women's experience

Having a positive smear puts women in a very vulnerable position. In particular, as I have already pointed out, it makes us stop and think about things, and so naturally about our sexual, intimate relationships. Of the women I talked to, a minority felt that their partners had no place in what was happening, and that this was their own experience, to be gone through alone. Most of them saw it as an experience that involved their partner; some saw it as an issue between their partner and themselves.

Abandonment

Very many women felt sad and angry at the way their partners reacted to their condition. The cry again and again was: 'My partner didn't seem to realize what I was going through.' We are talking here about the way partners behaved – and the fact that it was often not what women wanted. Here are some sample complaints: 'My partner . . . was away all the time . . . needed me for comfort . . . didn't believe how serious it was . . . didn't want to know . . . didn't want to talk about it . . . built a brick wall . . . refused to read any of the literature . . . didn't come with me to the hospital and that finished our relationship.'

It was not all negative. There were also many women who said their partners were supportive and gave them what they needed. Many of the women quoted above had stable relationships that in other ways were totally satisfactory. Some women, in fact, wanted less support, not more, as it made them feel dependent and weak to be over-protected.

However there did seem to be a pattern of male partners in particular seemingly 'not understanding . . . listening . . . taking it seriously.' If you feel that this is your partner's response, you are not alone. It does not mean that your relationship is at an end – as we shall see when we look at the other side of the story, it doesn't even mean that your partner doesn't understand you. Nevertheless, you may start to panic, feeling that just at the time when you need support most, your partner is not there for you. As we shall see later, you may well be right – but not for the reasons that you suspect.

Blame

'Often, when you hear that you have a positive smear, your first thought is: Who did I get this from?' as one woman put it. At the time of going to press, the link between sexual contact and cervical cancer is not clear, nor is it proven. Equally, it may not be the particular trigger that made you vulnerable. It is newsworthy, however, and sufficiently publicized for many women immediately to jump to the conclusion that they 'caught' their cervical condition from a man.

Many women made this connection, and spoke scathingly of partners because of it. Some blamed past partners: 'We split up two and a half years ago . . . I feel this [the CIN condition] is the result of him having other relationships which I hadn't known about at the time,' said Rosemary. Some blamed present partners: 'The first thing I said when I heard was, "I'll kill him",' said one woman. Some women felt confused and uncertain: 'I don't blame him – but I want to know what caused it,' said Linda.

For lesbian women in particular, such a cause and effect link may create added problems. For those who have previously had heterosexual relationships, the memories of these relationships may be particularly painful, and the addition of blame for a current disease adds insult to injury.

Many women, of course, saw the male-female link as absolutely not a problem. 'We didn't enter into that,' said Julie, 'I know that isn't an issue for us . . .' They knew that there was a possibility of a kickback from previous relationships, but it wasn't relevant to their present security. In any case, as one woman said, 'I've also had relationships before ours; it might have been me rather than him.'

It is totally understandable that if a past or present partner has passed a medical problem on to you, you should be upset by this. It is not a pleasant thing to have. Mary, who caught the wart virus from her boyfriend, was 'very angry as well as hurt'. And if your partner does have an infection or virus and is unwilling to have it treated, then you are right to be angry. It is also understandable if you are hurt by your partner's past and present sexual history. If we are not the only sexual partner in our partner's life, then that may also provoke strong feeling. So if your cervical condition reminds you of the fact that your male partner has slept with other women, then don't be surprised if you start to feel negative. Equally, if your cervical condition reminds your female partner that you have in the past slept with men, you may have to cope with that.

Remember, however, that it is never certain that your partner's past or present sexual history has any direct link with your particular current condition. Many women have relationships with men without developing cervical cancer, while some women who have never had a heterosexual relationship will develop cervical conditions. There are many vulnerability factors that can band together to affect you, of which sexually-caused vulnerability is only one.

Positive Smear

Political anger

Some women who spoke to me placed the responsibility on men in a much wider sense. They felt that men in general were to blame for irresponsible sexual behaviour which might be spreading the 'cancer trigger'. They felt that in the arena of sexual politics, men were the oppressors again by inflicting yet another sexual disease on women.

Arguments for and against the 'cancer trigger' theory apart, it seems to be a big leap of judgment to say that men are therefore to blame for cervical cancer. Certainly if there is a direct link between sexual activity and cervical abnormality, the current tendency to blame women is not the answer. Yet neither, I think, is blaming men. Men should assume equal responsibility for taking precautions, not only against cervical cancer but against all forms of sexually transmitted disease, as well as against pregnancy. Men, like women, should guard against these things by being responsible in safe sex, and by working to enhance and prolong good, fulfilling relationships.

However, to say, as some people do while championing women's causes, that cervical cancer is men's fault, is too easy a route. If the cancer trigger is a virus, and a man has caught it, then who has he caught it from? It is more than likely that he has caught it from another woman, who in turn has caught it from a man, who in turn . . . If the 'cancer trigger' is not a virus, but is rogue sperm, then it is neither men's fault for having rogue sperm, nor women's fault for being attracted to men.

Guilt

If a male ex-partner of yours is now going out with someone new,

192

this can lead to further bad feelings. My ex-lover's new girlfriend developed CIN 2 and had laser treatment. I was tempted to believe that he had caught something from me and passed 'it' on to his new girlfriend – and that it was my fault.

If you are scared of this, and you have just had a positive smear result, then you may feel you ought to mention it to your ex-partner. But remember that it is up to him and his new partner to make their own decisions about what they do; whether they use barrier contraception, whether she goes for a smear test. It is their responsibility. Remember that, as Jacqui said, 'She's seen the programmes just the same as I have.' If it is sexually transmitted, then she is as likely to have caught it from a former partner as from anything you have passed on to her through him.

Lack of sexual interest

Sadly, quite a few women I talked to spoke of general effects on their attitudes to sex, and therefore on their intimate relationships.

'I just went off sex because I had so many internals,' said Heather. 'I don't think we've had a normal sex life since it happened because every time we have intercourse, I bleed,' said Anna. While Linda commented, 'I wouldn't bother if I never had "it" again . . .'

It is sad that this happens. When your feelings about your cervix are altered, by examinations, treatment and the suggestions of a link between disease and your sex life, then your sexuality may well be affected. But it needn't be like this. With more consideration and support from the very beginning, from medical and lay people alike, maybe you can begin to realize that you can separate your cervix from your sexuality – so that one remains intact even if the other is going through a vulnerable time. Some women, in fact, felt that particularly after their treatment, beginning to make love again was part of the healing process.

Partners' experience – the men

I spoke to a number of men whose partners had had a positive smear, CIN or cancer. I began by being fairly negative – I had heard so many complaints of men 'not understanding' or 'not listening'. But as the interviews progressed, I realized that what I was hearing was not evidence of male unfeelingness. If anything it was the opposite. What I was hearing was about men who were almost as deeply touched by the experience as their partners were.

Fear or knowledge?

An overriding emotion that many men feel when their partner is ill is fear. And just as we as women are confused and afraid, so can men be. They too can be unsure whether you have cancer or not. Are you going to die? Are they going to lose their partner?

This fear can paralyse. Many women spoke of husbands who could not and would not admit what their condition was: 'I don't think he believed it until we learned I had to have a hysterectomy,' said Diana of her husband. 'He got into his research to a ridiculous extent . . . I realized afterwards that it was because he was worried,' said Heather of her boyfriend.

Even when it becomes clear that your CIN condition is not going to be fatal, your partner may still be frightened. Alain spoke of his real fear that Emma, his wife, might be seriously ill, even though her condition was only CIN 2. 'I burst into tears saying, "Emma might die, Emma might die." '

Remember too that in just the same way as your past experiences have affected your attitude to illness and death, so your partner's past experiences have affected his. Judith's boyfriend had nearly died after a bike accident: 'He thought I was dying, the whole time – and after what he'd been through, he couldn't handle it.' Heather's partner Cedric remembered his grandparents dying of cancer and he was 'very scared'.

Men's fear can come out in different ways from women's fear, because of the different ways we have been brought up. A man may feel uneasy at showing fear, and choose instead to ignore the emotion. He may be angry, he may just deny it is happening, or belittle your illness. 'After all, you haven't got cancer,' Linda's husband said. He may feel that if he gives in to his fear, he will lose face, or be unable to help you with yours.

Just as with women, information can help men to overcome the fear. If a man is informed from the beginning about what is going on and is involved in what is happening, then he will know as much as you will, and will be able to make his own judgments about how serious your condition is. He will be less confused about what CIN means and what it means for you. Many women reported that their partners discussed the hospital leaflets with them, and made great efforts to understand the various stages.

195

Positive Smear

If your condition is serious, and you can talk about this together, then both your fears will find an outlet: 'We did talk seriously about what would happen if I died . . .' said Diana. 'When we heard the news, we talked all night . . . we realized that we'd been very lucky,' said Sue.

Exclusion or involvement?

Men can feel very excluded from what is happening. A man's previous experience of 'women's plumbing problems', as one man sarcastically described his fellow men's approach to things, may have been minimal. And if men don't have the benefit of reading the information, chatting to informed women friends, or facing the medical professionals themselves, then they may well feel excluded and powerless: 'Someone else was helping Heather a lot, and I found this really threatening. I felt inadequate,' said Cedric. 'It was something to do with her body, not with mine,' said Ian.

Many women complained that men didn't get involved – and particularly that they didn't come to hospital appointments as support. If a man, for whatever reason, doesn't feel able to do this – perhaps because he feels he will be in the way – then a vicious circle is created. The more he backs off from involvement, the more he will feel excluded and the less confident he will be.

Some men are able to involve themselves in what is happening. Andrew 'went through all the leaflets with Rachel, discussing what things meant'. Cedric set out to get photocopies of medical articles for his partner to read. Many men were present while their partners had outpatients'

196

treatment, literally holding their hands and giving them support. And the women appreciated this: 'It was really good having him there,' said one woman. 'It made me feel as if we were doing it together.'

Another way in which men can be involved might be to step back from what is happening and leave women to find their own power: 'I was put in a situation where, as Emma's best friend, she wanted me to help her decide whether to have treatment or not . . . but it was such an important decision that I couldn't really be involved in it.' This kind of attitude can seem too objective – but Emma did make her own decision, and was thankful to Alain for letting her make it alone.

Blame or support?

If men are aware of recent press coverage of cervical conditions, then they may feel blamed. If a woman feels that her partner is to blame, then he will certainly feel blamed. 'I know you blame me for it,' said Linda's husband to her – and this reaction was echoed in a number of other accounts.

Whether a man has some cause to feel guilty or not, being blamed may cause him to feel guilty – and angry and resentful. I understand this; we women felt angry and resentful not so long ago when all the blame was being put on us. And if a man cares for his partner, he may feel very threatened by the thought that he has harmed her. As he reacts angrily, she may feel equally threatened, and a cycle of resentment may build up.

So this is one area where men and women can actually ease each other's unhappiness. If the woman doesn't feel bitter, this will allow the man to be more at ease. When I was interviewing Rachel and Andrew, I touched on the question of blame, to be met by genuinely relaxed smiles: 'Well, we talked about that but . . .' It was very obvious that it wasn't an issue for Andrew – because it wasn't an issue for Rachel.

Frustration or acceptance?

Several women reported to me that their husbands were very understanding, until it came to the matter of sex. Men may be angry or frustrated at not being able to make love after their partner's treatment, or at having the spontaneity of sex removed by a change to barrier contraception. There is no reason for either partner to be angry because the other partner will not make love, but as one woman commented wryly, 'My husband's been without for six months, and in normal circumstances he could divorce me for that.'

Particularly if the experience has been bad for you, and you do not feel like making love for a long while, tempers may get frayed. Perhaps for the first time in your relationship, you may need to say 'no' to sex, so that you have time to heal, in every sense of the word. Some women coped with this in their own way. Some were able to make a distinction between love-making with penetration, which they didn't want, and love-making with masturbation, which they felt more at ease with – though as one woman commented to me: 'We didn't get married just to masturbate.'

There are other ways of coping. Viki, at the start of a new relationship, postponed her treatment for two weeks so that she and her new partner could enjoy love-making and stabilize their relationship: 'When the doctor said, "No sex for six weeks," I thought: This is going to wreck it – but I shouldn't have worried as much as I did since my partner was very good and supportive.'

Some women just stated their needs and had them met: 'I went home and said to [my partner], "That's it – from now on you use a condom."' For others of us, who have not been so assertive throughout our relationship, it is difficult suddenly to ask for what we need. And in the area of sex, particularly, we and our men may feel uncomfortable. Many of the men I spoke to had been accepting and supportive, however. Some were happy to wait until their partners felt good about penetrative sex, others spontaneously suggested using barrier contraception: 'He's been very good – we've just got closer and closer, even though we haven't had a normal sex life since it happened,' said Anna.

Independence or vulnerability?

More than one man admitted to needing support – and feeling uneasy about this. For so often, the role men are expected to play in our society is one of supporting the woman. Julie's partner 'seemed to feel he had to be "really strong and manly and I'm here if you want me", rather than dealing with his own feelings about it.'

To complicate matters further, a man may feel that his own need for support should take second place. As Cedric said, 'How can you justify wanting your own support system when your partner hasn't got one? You feel you have to bear it alone.' Many men had found their own way out, by confiding in friends about what was happening. But many are not used to asking for and receiving support, and may not have ready-made support networks.

It is by no means always appropriate for a man to ask his partner for comfort when her condition is serious. Sue's husband's way of coping with her hysterectomy was to tell her constantly, 'Well of course I'm upset about it too,' until one day she lost her temper with him: 'I'm sick and tired of comforting you . . .'. She felt better about it, and he learned something from that. But, sometimes if your partner can admit his vulnerability and you can accept it, that alone will enhance your relationship enormously. 'It's just getting better and better,' as one woman said.

Men's experience – what is going on?

The overwhelming impression I got of men both through their own accounts and those of their partners was that they did not mean to hurt women, but did so – unintentionally.

Many men were feeling confused and afraid, threatened and blamed, and reacted by being defensive. They usually shut off their emotions, and retreated into their heads, either because this was the way they were all the time, or because they felt they could not cope. It was not that they didn't realize the seriousness of the situation that made them like this. It was because they *did* appreciate its seriousness and were unable to deal with the implications, while at the same time being 'strong' for their partner. They often admitted to feeling very negative about themselves.

This may not ring true for you. I did hear stories of men

behaving in ways which were obviously not motivated by concern: 'I suspect one or two of the girls have had hidings from their husbands over this . . .' was the knowing comment of a woman from a support group in Liverpool. You may, however, like to consider the possibility that where your partner is not able to give you what you want, it is because he is too upset, rather than not upset enough.

Partners' experience – the women

Female partners have a slightly different set of issues to cope with. Where problems can arise is in the area of blame. A positive smear can raise all kinds of spectres of previous heterosexual relationships, on both sides. A woman already threatened by her lover's male ex-partners, may feel both fear and anger against men in general and against the particular man whose actions seem to have made the woman she loves ill. Also, the question of fidelity may be raised: 'you didn't catch it from me . . . who did you catch it from?'

Conversely, lesbian partnerships may be in a much stronger position to offer mutual support. A woman partner may be able to respond positively to news of an abnormal smear simply because she can imagine what that feels like better than a man can. Perhaps she has had one too; at any rate, she knows that she too is at risk. She often feels able to read the information leaflets with her partner, to overcome fear with real knowledge and personal insight. She is far less tempted to exclude herself from what is happening and far less likely to be excluded, because she is a woman too. 'My partner made me feel that there were two of us going through the whole thing – because she shared it with me', said Jan.

So what do we do?

We've looked at things that can go wrong for women in an intimate relationship. We've looked at partners' experiences. Often, just being aware of these can help (even if it means you leave this book open at an appropriate page for him/her to read).

Let's end the chapter with a positive statement of what it could be like, based on what people I interviewed said they wanted and had often managed to obtain. In what ways can two people in an intimate relationship work together to make the experience a positive one?

Firstly, it could be the chance really to communicate and talk things through. Many couples said that the shock had forced them to do this, and that after the event they had 'kept on talking'. Secondly, you could learn much about each other's needs when under stress: 'I actually needed space to deal with it on my own . . .' said Julie. 'I needed him to come to the hospital with me,' said Rosemary. 'We went, as women together, to face it together,' said Amy.

You may be able to learn to allow the other person to have their feelings, unimpeded by criticism. Anna comments: 'My partner was great; he never said it's OK, he always said, "it's awful" – and that really helped me because that was what I was feeling too.'

It can be a time of amazingly close physical support; many couples found themselves hugging more than usual, even though their desire to make love was diminished. It can be comforting to know that you don't need to make love in order to be close to each other.

On the practical side, as a heterosexual couple, you might learn to use barrier contraception for both your sakes. You might find out you can create intimate relationships that are no less intimate, and no less spontaneous for being risk-free – and that barrier contraception can be a telling sign of what you feel for each other, and how much you care and want to protect each other.

You can get really close by tackling the system together, by going together to examinations, fighting for the treatment you want. You can look back and think: 'We survived that together,' and feel closer because of it.

13   The professionals

*‘ In terms of the treatment I got,
I'm satisfied. In terms of the
attitude of the consultant, I'm
not. ’*
(Frances)

As soon as you enter the system, you come face to face with the professionals. From the moment you have the smear test, through the result, the diagnosis and the treatment, they are there. They guide you, help you and sometimes hinder you. How can you make the best out of this necessary relationship? How can you turn it into a positive meeting of equals that gets you back to health as soon as possible?

Who are the professionals?

Most of the medical professionals we meet fall into three groups. First are the GPs or local clinic doctors. They are usually the ones who break the news of a positive smear to us and suggest the next step. And some of the stories I heard about them were wonderful. Julie's direct question of her doctor: 'Have I got cancer?' was answered equally directly with a: 'No, you haven't', which strengthened her for her treatment and cure.

Next, we come into contact with nurses. They are present during our examination, diagnosis, and treatment. Their role is a little different. As we shall see, this makes a big difference to the way we can use them in our attempt to be actively involved in the situation. Most nurses don't make diagnoses or suggest treatment. They may take our original smear; they may offer us counselling before and after examination or treatment. They may support doctors in practical ways and patients in emotional ways. In current medical practice, the nurse is there as your representative in the system – your advocate to the doctor 'The nurse was marvellous – she held my hand and kept telling me irrelevant things to take my mind off the treatment,' said one woman.

Finally, we meet the consultant, be it a man or a woman. S/he uses his/her expertise to look, think, pronounce. We know that this person has experience and training. We may feel in awe of them, and we are certainly dependent on them in many ways for the treatment that will give us back our health. Many consultants add to this service by offering the best kind of professional interaction: by being supportive, objective, consultative. 'I really trusted my consultant,' said Rachel. 'He told me the truth.'

What goes right?

At its best, the system works very well. The medical

professionals are trained and experienced and they do their job. They take account of your body and your mental state, and work to heal both. There has been a dramatic drop in the death rate for invasive cervical cancer over the last ten years. In the stories I heard in my original research for the book, there was example after example of good treatment, of problems spotted in time, of diagnoses carefully made, of survival of even the worst problems. One doctor tried to get therapy on the NHS for a patient who hated internal examination. Another 'gave me any amount of time. I could have sat in that room for ever and he wouldn't have minded,' said Rachel. One London GP, Jane Chomet, had even installed a colposcope in her surgery, an example to us all of her commitment to her patients.

Since this book was first published, some extraordinarily positive developments have occurred. The system, in general, has begun to provide a much better service: regular screening, organized recall, quality control for smear tests. Individual medical professionals have often shifted their attitudes to understand the patient's viewpoint in a way they never did before. Many have seen the need for further information, and have written leaflets and even books designed to fill that information gap. Many have pushed for counselling facilities for their patients, gone on counselling courses themselves, set up training so that others can learn to counsel.

Particularly impressive is the way they have invited patients into the system, to bridge the gap and enable learning on both sides. I asked, in the first edition of this book, for an opportunity to let patients talk to consultants about how it feels to be treated. This has already begun to happen. I personally have spoken on many a course about this book and its message; Lily spends a lot of her time talking to consultants about 'the patients' point of view'; following her personal experience of hysterectomy, Vivienne was invited to work at her local colposcopy clinic to help improve services.

The Positive Smear Conference Update Report[23, 24] showed 'a great improvement... much more client-professional equality... we are much more aware of the trauma now... we allow a longer period of time to discuss client anxiety... most patients are counselled now... we leave a phone number for them to ring if they feel the need... we give more information... books... videos... leaflets... I am now doing a regular programme on community radio'. All in all, we have to say that there has been a positive response from professionals to women with positive smears.

What goes wrong?

With the system

Despite all this optimism, the feeling of many women involved in my original writing of this book is still echoed by women today – that the system, the medical health care machine, often does not respond in the best way possible. The resources are not there to make it what it could be. Many of these complaints don't just apply to cervical illnesses or to gynaecological Outpatients wards – but nevertheless, complaints there are.

Firstly of course, there are not enough resources put into screening services. 'Every five years' say the recommendations, mainly because 'every three years' would put a strain on already tightly stretched resources – a fact that even the doctors' own screening guidelines now admit. Medical professionals, having now accepted that there is a need, find themselves frustrated because there is no money to meet that need: for smears done more quickly, for information material, for counsellors, for training, for research.

There is still, too, a seeming lack of care and thought in the system, also no doubt because lack of funds leaves little time for luxuries. The letter you are sent inviting you for a smear, or asking you back for colposcopy, can be impersonal and badly produced. Information may not be given before, during or after your treatment. The waiting list for examination can be months and once there, you often have to wait hours in the waiting room: 'I waited until one o'clock for a ten o'clock appointment,' said one woman. When at last your turn comes, nurses are often rushing from one place to another and have no time to spend with you. Often the procedures for undressing make you feel vulnerable or uncomfortable. In the consulting room, the same is often true. Doctors have obviously seen many more patients than their energy and attention is up to. They are as exhausted and stressed as you are. Usually, you don't see the same doctors and nurses every time you attend: 'I went six times and saw someone different on every occasion,' said one woman.

The waiting list for treatment may be just as long as that for diagnosis, and when treatment is given, there may not be counselling facilities to support you before the experience or, in Outpatients, the facilities to sit down afterwards, to have a cup of tea, to have a hug from your friend or partner, to recover your breath. As an inpatient, too, you can feel as if you were on a conveyor belt, as overworked nurses shunt you through to make room for tomorrow morning's batch.

In addition, the system has, it seems, thrown up two new problems that are not to do with resources. The Government's new screening system, which asks GPs to recall their patients regularly, in order to gain a funding allowance, is a real move to offer screening to all women in the UK. But perhaps this pressure on GPs to reach a certain quota of patient smears may lead in turn to GPs pressurizing patients. We have already had examples of doctors removing patients from their register because those patients would not accept their due smear test.[25] This seems to me misguided; we are, of course, looking for all women to accept screening, but by taking the decision out of their hands, and penalizing them for not accepting, we are surely, in the short-term, disempowering them, and making it less likely that in the long-term women will take responsibility for their own health.

A second cause for worry concerns treatment. It has become apparent over the last few years that many mild cervical conditions get better on their own, without treatment, yet many doctors will push for the treatment option. This could be because it is cheaper to treat (one or two visits) than to monitor (several six-monthly checks) or it may reflect the general preference of doctors and most patients. As women with CIN1, we can resist pressure to accept treatment, choosing to return rather than be treated right away, but the fact remains that professionals may not be able to offer this option easily and happily.

The bottom line on all these issues is that they are rarely the fault of individuals; they stem directly from the system, the way it works and the way it allocates its resources. But they are a problem and they do need to be recognized, challenged and, as soon as possible, changed.

With the people

In the course of writing this book I found ample evidence of professional and competent conduct, skill and sensitivity, but I was left with the disturbing overall impression that there still seems to be something wrong.

During my original research, I interviewed over thirty women who had had positive smears, and many of their relatives, and received written statements from more. During the years since the book, and particularly as a result of the Update Report, I heard from many other patients and professionals too. As I collected information, it became apparent that the dominant feeling was one of concern. Women had been seen, diagnosed and treated successfully; that was, on the whole, not where concern lay. What seems at issue was not the treatment, but the way in which women were being treated, and this concern came from patients and professionals alike.

I include this preamble because I am not simply using one or two hysterical complaints to make a statement about women's needs. I am, I think, reflecting what many women feel about the way the medical profession reacts to cervical conditions. I am undoubtedly sticking my neck out, but perhaps this will help to change current attitudes.

There were a number of ways in which women thought that they could have been treated better.

211

Positive Smear

The first general complaint was that there was little equal personal contact. Women asked for 'eye contact as I walked in', 'some words aimed at me, not just at the other doctor', 'a response to questions I asked, please'. Others would have appreciated more delicacy: 'Don't walk in on me while I'm undressing,' was one plea. 'I just felt like another pair of spread legs, another piece of research,' commented another woman. These were all appeals for equality, for being treated like another adult with a need for respect. Although this cry is frequently heard in other medical contexts, in this area women perhaps have a more pronounced need.

Some women felt blamed by medical professionals. This is more often due to unfeeling media hype than doctors actually accusing patients face to face, but any number of articles in the medical press contain attacks on women's behaviour. 'Dr X blames permissiveness, promiscuity and the copulation explosion,' reads one quote from *The Times*, the speaker an eminent British gynaecologist. It continues, 'I am aware that it might be rather futile advice, but if young women refrained from sex until they were in their twenties . . .' Such statements can only give women the impression that the medical profession is critical of them.

Medical professionals could be more careful, too, about assuming that cervical conditions have been sexually transmitted (as we know, the evidence is not clear), and about assuming that a patient is heterosexual at all (sometimes she isn't). They could also try giving messages about sexual care and protection without 'telling off'. Advice about contraception is one thing; emotional pressure to adopt specific methods of contraception is another. 'I don't need to be told I must,' said one woman, 'I just want to be told what the options are'.

When it comes to giving information about the options, things could also improve. Women who do need the information (there are some, in fact, who would prefer not to know, and their preference should be respected)[26], want it given sensitively, simply and with no jargon, clearly and with honesty. They want professionals not to hang on to knowledge, taking a monopoly on expertise; they want knowledge shared so that, aware of what their medical situation is, each woman can make her own health choices.

Another worry women had was the powerlessness they felt when confronted by medical professionals. They had frequently felt excluded from any involvement in their cases and this had been manifested in a number of ways – for example, in the refusal of doctors to give patients information: 'My doctor would not give me my smear result – in the end I went back with my sister and demanded a repeat smear,' said Heather. Few doctors really discussed with patients what was happening, or presented options for treatment. There were, as I have mentioned previously, several cases of patients seeking second opinions to get the treatment they felt was appropriate. And there was also a feeling among women that doctors in general had a vested interest in appearing infallible.

A final thought. Many of the women I spoke to had also had other medical treatment in the past about which they rarely spoke with such concern. It does appear that cervical-related illness is an area which causes women to feel particularly vulnerable, or in which professionals display a particular lack of sensitivity. I am not the first writer to suggest that specializing in gynaecology can be linked with feelings of power in doctors. And perhaps cervical cancer and CIN, where sexuality is so closely linked with disease, is more of a minefield than many other diseases. Dare I suggest that in this area, particularly, doctors may themselves feel ill at ease and unable to communicate with patients, and it is this which causes dissatisfaction on the part of so many patients?

The professionals' point of view

Of course, no argument is ever one-sided. There are reasons to be sympathetic towards the medical profession, and it has to be appreciated that what we as women experience is often not what the professionals *want* us to feel.

Doctors and nurses are only human; they are frequently overworked and some, particularly the nurses, are drastically underpaid. They work in a very stressful environment. The many professionals I talked to were all extremely committed to eradicating cancer and the stages leading up to it. Most of them were depressed by the unceasing stream of women with cervical conditions that poured through their surgeries and consulting rooms for treatment.

I can understand then the angry frustration of a doctor who thinks he has tracked down a cause and wants people to listen, or the inability of a nurse to keep her patience when there is a three-hour backlog in the waiting-room. I can also understand the unease of doctors who are not resolved in their own minds about sexuality and its place in their lives, having to treat women whose very condition is a reminder of sexuality.

Sometimes, particularly with minor CIN conditions, it must be difficult to remember that to the patient, this is a serious matter. It can be hard to understand the emotion of a woman with CIN1 when the last patient you treated had advanced invasive cancer. Sometimes, too, it must be easy to forget that you are not God when you are making life and death decisions all day and every day.

Medical professionals, like everyone else, are the product of a society that undervalues women. As someone commented: 'If 2,000 men a year died of cancer of the testicles, there would be an outcry.' So perhaps we should understand when women are treated lightly in a medical situation – this is, after all, only a reflection of what happens in the outside world.

I can also imagine many people reading this and thinking that the women I interviewed were biased. After all, they saw the doctor at a time when they were both vulnerable and ill. This is certainly at the heart of the matter. Women are, as one consultant said, 'vulnerable, probably frightened and probably going to be in some discomfort'. But this is, to me, not evidence that women are biased. It is evidence that there needs to be a rethink. Someone needs to get the message through to everyone concerned that it is at this time that women are most in need of care and sensitive handling.

Blame or change?

I have read articles that attack medical attitudes in a far stronger way than I am doing here. This is because I think it is a waste of energy to blame. To quote Lily Hopkins, also a fighter for positive smear change, 'My battle is not *against* anybody. It is a battle *for* lives.' I would rather use that energy to change. It is my feeling that unless we are all prepared to take responsibility for changing what seems to be happening, then nothing will change. It is hard to expect women to try to

215

change a system when what they are really concerned about is getting themselves better. This is why on many occasions, I suggest taking a supporter or friend with you.

The fact remains that however hard people on the outside try, it is only when people in the system start taking action that attitudes will change. If we as patients can begin to expect to be treated as competent equals, then maybe we will be.

What can we do?

As patients

There are lots of practical things we can do to move into a position where we and medical professionals can work together to create health. Many of these have been mentioned in the book where they are relevant, but here is a summary:

The first thing we can do is to make sure that on a physical level we are not vulnerable. We can in a general sense take responsibility for our own health, take preventative measures, turn up for regular smear tests, and for treatment when it is necessary. When we do so, as I have mentioned elsewhere, it is possible and usual now in most hospitals to be examined without undressing, to insist on taking a friend in with you for support, and to ask for the physical help you need, such as local anaesthetic. Some treatments are uncomfortable and some are painful, but as far as you can, take care of your own physical needs, and you will feel more in charge.

The second thing is that we need to become knowledgeable.

216

Knowledge is the doctor's speciality; but if we are able to listen with understanding and ask questions based on that understanding, then we are beginning to be equal. The Facts section of this book contains some of the basics, and throughout the book I suggest questions to ask your doctor.

You can ask to be shown your records, and told about your diagnosis and treatment, if you want to. You do have the choice, though this means you also have the responsibility. You can ask the doctor why s/he is recommending a particular treatment, ask what would happen if other treatments were used, challenge the suggestion that you be treated immediately if you would rather wait and, in general discuss your fears and concerns with staff.

You can also turn to the nurses for help. They are usually women, and may even have had a positive smear themselves. Current nurses' training teaches that the nurse is an 'advocate' on your behalf. In a fascinating interview with a representative of the Royal College of Nursing, I learnt that 'the patient has personal power, but the nurse has power in the system . . . to plead for the patient.'

A distance will always exist between medical professionals and their patients. Without this protective measure, many doctors would be powerless to help us, because they would be far too involved. But in the case of nurses, the system is organized in such a way that they have the power to support us. Remember, then, that if you feel unsupported, and if you feel powerless, it is not you that is at fault. It means that the system is breaking down.

If all else fails, you can complain about treatment. Your Community Health Council will advise you on your rights and support you in writing to the appropriate body; you will find their number in your phone book.

217

Positive Smear

It is not possible to change the attitudes of all doctors overnight. If you suddenly start questioning and arguing, professionals who have never been questioned in their lives may react negatively. You may be afraid (two or three women were) that if you argue, you will get worse treatment. So don't push yourself beyond your limits.

In taking equal responsibility it must, of course, be borne in mind that once we do, our health is up to us. So if we are going to act as equals, we should take care of ourselves by going for regular smears, taking exercise and eating good food, working with the treatment we decide on and not against it. It's a long-term responsibility and it isn't an easy one.

As non-patients

Whether we are patients or not, we can still improve the system. Partners, whether male or female, can help. They can stand beside positive smear women and fight the system when it blocks progress in general, and the specific progress of individual women on their way to regaining health. Often, the positive smear woman herself is too caught up in her illness to challenge the system, whereas a partner has the energy to make the phone calls, pressure the administration, make a fuss.

And, even when not directly affected, everyone can fight for better professional conditions. Joining pressure groups, raising money for better hospital equipment, pushing for counselling facilities – these things can be done by ordinary lay people. Inspired by the death from cervical cancer of an ordinary member of the community, people in my town formed a committee that has almost single-handedly kept the local colposcopy clinic funded: the Myrtle Peach Trust now continues to raise money through charity events to buy other hospital equipment.

As professionals

Let me first say that I am aware of the pressures medical professionals are under, and the limitations and lack of resources under which they constantly work.

I am also grateful. Doctors and nurses have saved my life on three occasions, and many of those I have known and met have been wonderful. I also know that a large number of medical professionals who will read this book are innocent of any of the charges I have levelled in this chapter. I'm also aware that a list of things to do won't change anything. Only altering attitudes does that.

But nevertheless, there are some things that medical professionals could fight for, for everyone's sake. They could, for instance, continue to fight within the system for the money and the resources to give more help to positive smear women.

How could this be used? In so many ways. It would be wonderful to get faster reporting on smears, more spotting of errors in smear readings, to whittle down waiting lists for diagnosis and for treatment, to buy more effective equipment, to provide helpful leaflets to inform women, to provide support services to build health before and after treatment.

In one clinic I heard about, there were pictures on the ceiling and music playing while women were being treated – a result of action taken by the staff working there. Could we also

Positive Smear

have professionals fighting to spend more time with each patient, to give more information and involve her more fully in the process?

How about a counsellor on hand, after examination, diagnosis, treatment? How about a counsellor on hand to counsel both partners if evidence of the wart virus has been found? How about help directly for the professionals: more research into the causes, the treatments, the psychology, so that they could build their medical practice on even more solid ground? Why not give them more training, particularly in counselling skills, and more opportunities for networking, for colleague contact, for interdepartmental liaison, so that they felt supported as they worked?

Finally, I shall just ask any medical professionals to do two things: firstly, read this book with an open mind; secondly, the next time you meet a woman with a positive smear condition, and you ask her 'How are you?', stop and wait for the answer, the real answer.

220

14 Some personal stories

During the course of writing and revising this book, I interviewed over sixty people and received written accounts or resource material from some thirty more. Of the sixty, over half were women who have had a positive smear, with consequences ranging from no treatment through to radical hysterectomy. Although a large proportion of the ideas, thoughts and examples I have given throughout the book are taken from these women's accounts, I also thought it would be useful to include some more detailed accounts of what happened.

I have chosen these four experiences not because they are dramatic or moving – although they certainly are that. I have chosen them because each, in its own way, is typical of the experiences women related to me. In these four accounts, the main issues – fears, doubts, problems, concerns – of the women I interviewed, are all reflected.

Positive Smear

I have edited the original interviews so that they read more or less chronologically and in an ordered way; these edits have been checked and approved by the interviewees. Occasionally, to introduce a topic, I have added an introductory phrase or two; these are always indicated in square brackets. Otherwise these words, thoughts and feelings are the women's own.

Rosemary

I was supposed to have had a smear test in May, and in fact I went in June. I got the letter back very quickly saying come and see us immediately. Then I rushed off to the Family Planning doctor, then to the hospital with the hot little note in my hand, and then of course it just disappeared into the system.

I panicked after a while because I hadn't heard anything about an appointment, and I phoned them up. They said, 'Oh, it's all right. The reason you haven't had an appointment yet is because the consultant doesn't think your case is really urgent – otherwise you'd have been in here by now.' Why didn't they tell me instead of leaving me waiting?

My immediate reaction when I heard the news was sheer terror. I didn't want to talk about it at all. I kept thinking: 'Oh God, I'm going to die. What will happen to the children?' I'm not someone who usually panics, but it was so unexpected.

I had a colposcopy and then laser treatment a few months later. It is actually painless, not an unpleasant experience at all, very quick, and the doctors and nurses were very sweet and charming. It was a woman who did the treatment, and she was super, although I have this feeling that if you're older, like I am, they treat you better. But I felt quite sad during it, which I hadn't expected at all. I don't see why it wasn't like giving a pint of blood, even less than that, . . . but it wasn't.

After the treatment, I had intended to go and buy a compost bin. But the friend who came with me, who had had laser treatment before I did, told me to go home instead. I did, and I was glad I did, because I did feel funny, though I don't know why. I wonder whether it was the local anaesthetic? I didn't feel cramps, at least not until later, and I had some bleeding but not much.

[Why do I think I got it?] My doctor said it was the wart virus, and at first I thought: 'Oh that's nothing.' But when my friend explained to me what she'd heard about the wart virus, and what it can do, I was really very shocked. It created real problems for me.

My husband had left about two-and-a-half years ago, and I felt that he was to blame, because he'd had other relationships. I really felt that it was some sort of venereal disease. It's unfair to blame him, because it takes two people to get anything, but I did.

I also felt very worried that I'd had a short sexual affair with somebody who is married, as a real fling when my husband first went off, and I wondered whether I should write and tell this man. The thought of his picking up something from me and giving it to his wife was really quite frightening. I did try to talk to my husband about it a bit, but I probably handled it totally wrongly because I felt quite angry . . . it's quite a difficult thing to talk to somebody about . . .

So when I had to go for treatment, I felt I didn't want any relationships any more. I feel the whole thing is bound up with many areas of your life, not just ones about the cervix.

I think it's changed my attitude to sex in relation to my

daughters too. I didn't tell my younger daughter, but I did talk to the older one about it all, though I don't want her to be anxious about it. I hope she avoids going to bed with people early in her life – she's thirteen now.

What I'm left with is a feeling that having a positive smear is a lot like childbirth. It's sexual, it's medical. There are things you can confide in someone who has been through it that you wouldn't confide in someone who hasn't. And it gets to every bit of you . . . you have got to come to terms with the relationship you're having, what's happened to it, your own mortality . . . I think there are a lot of similarities.

Frances

The first time I realized that something was wrong was when I started bleeding after intercourse. It was a good enough excuse for me to go down to the Family Planning Clinic, and they did a smear there, which my GP had never done.

First of all they said I had an erosion on my cervix, which would heal on its own. The bleeding went on for the best part of a year and it got to the stage where I was getting agitated.

Then they sent me to the colposcopy clinic. They did some tests and said there were some pre-cancerous cells and that it would be dealt with by laser treatment at Outpatients.

When I first heard, I did panic. You have great fears of: 'Oh God, my grandmother died of cancer of the womb. Is it hereditary?' Outwardly there wasn't a lot of change really, although I lost a lot of weight. Inwardly though I lost confidence and in some ways I haven't really got it all back. I don't seem to take the initiative; I just seem to draw into myself a lot of the time.

I also wondered what caused it. It seems that they just don't know. I've kept asking them: 'Is it the Pill that's causing it?' because I've been on the Pill for twelve years and it's probably about time I came off it, what with my being overweight and smoking. But the doctor just says, 'No, you carry on with it.' I haven't found anything that explains particularly well why a positive smear happens. If they told me there was anything I should be doing, then I'd do it, and quite happily. But no one told me to do anything.

The question of how many partners I've had came from the doctor. When I went to the clinic, the doctor said, 'How active a sex life do you have? How many different boyfriends have you had?' as if my sleeping around was the cause of it. I was thinking: 'I've only ever had three boyfriends; is it that bad?'

There was never any question of that from my husband; I know he's had previous partners, he knows I have and I know one of his girlfriends quite well. There's never been any tension on either side about that.

[As for support] I don't suppose I really talked to my husband about it all. I managed to get him to come down to the hospital with me once, but he hates people being ill and can't cope with it. In other ways though he was quite good and understanding.

I haven't met anyone within my circle of friends who has suffered from it, or admits they have. So I doubt that I've told anyone except my sister. When I first had the treatment, she came to the hospital with me and stayed until Ian came home that evening, but other than that I haven't had any support as such.

Positive Smear

As for the doctors, in terms of the actual treatment I got, I'm quite satisfied with that. In terms of the attitude of the consultant, I'm not happy about that at all. I did get angry a few times and stood up for myself, and so that was positive.

[Support in terms of information?] I read round after the event but not before. I'm a library assistant – I first searched through our own stock to see if there was anything and there wasn't. There were odd references here and there but they were useless, far too technical.

When the time came to go for the laser treatment, I was frightened. They told me there wouldn't be any side effects, but that's not quite true. I took it easy, but we did go away for a walking trip afterwards, and by the time I got back four days later, I was absolutely exhausted.

My story hasn't really ended. After the first lot of treatment, I was still having the bleeding so they did a D&C. That was eighteen months ago. But it still hasn't been sorted out. I know something is still wrong.

Diana

I had three children and I was pregnant again. It was all planned. I was about thirteen weeks pregnant, and had a smear test, went back two or three weeks later and was told, 'You've got a positive smear, nothing to worry about. You'll be going to a colposcopy clinic, but it's OK.'

That night I came back absolutely fine, thinking there was nothing to worry about. I went to bed, woke up in the middle of the night and thought: 'My God, I'm dying.' It suddenly hit me that having a positive smear must mean that I had cancer.

226

I rang the hospital the next day and asked whether, if I had cancer, they would call me in immediately. They said of course they would, but when I came off the phone I just cried and cried all day. In the end my husband came home from work because I'd got myself into such a state about it.

When I went for my first examination, the doctor said he thought I would need treatment, but they would wait until I had the baby. There was never a point where I considered not having the baby, because by the time they spotted it, the baby was moving. At each consultation I remember saying to them, 'I've got to have a Caesarian; can't you do a hysterectomy at the same time?' And both the consultant and the registrar kept saying to me, 'You're jumping the gun. It won't come to that.'

My daughter was born in May, and after she was born, I just kept bleeding and was given tablets to stop it. I had my periods and in between 'spotting' practically every day. My fear was that it was an indication that things were more serious than a pre-cancer condition. I went back in September for a colposcopy and biopsy, and then for a cone biopsy. They took away 80 per cent of my cervix. The doctor was wonderful – he went specially to get the results for me and he told me that the results were good and that all the abnormal cells had been removed. I remember thinking: 'Well, this is wonderful. That's it. All over.'

I had a smear a month later which was fine, so by Christmas I thought everything was great. But then I started spotting again, and I went back for another smear and colposcopy.

Two weeks went by, and the doctor hadn't rung me. So I rang him. I asked him the result of my smear, and he said, 'I

227

can't remember.' And then I knew. The next day I got a phone call to say my smear was positive, and would I come in to see another doctor, this time with my husband.

We did that. She explained everything and then she said to me, 'You're thirty. You've had all your children. We think the best thing for you is to have a hysterectomy.' I came away thinking that the main reason to have a hysterectomy was to sterilize me, because of my age and the number of children I had. The doctor obviously found it hard to say that this treatment was necessary because of the abnormal smear. It preyed on my mind that this was not enough reason to have major surgery, so I wrote to the doctor saying I wouldn't have a hysterectomy. Then we saw another doctor who explained to me that in fact there were still abnormal cells in my cervix, in the canal. After that, my husband and I were both convinced that a hysterectomy was the only option, because, if left untreated, the cells would have become invasive cancer.

Then I went into the hospital to have the hysterectomy. I just let go and cried and cried and coped with it that way. The nurses were fantastic, the doctors would come and see me every day and let me ask questions over and over again until I understood. The experience was a positive one in that traumatic period of my life.

It was a hard time. I'm sure most people would feel that. I had been told that everything was clear, and then suddenly I was told that it had come back again. I did lose my trust. But it's all right now.

I did ask why it happened. The media says it is a sexually transmitted disease, and people just hear promiscuity. This was really brought home to me when my mother-in-law rang me one evening saying, 'I got talking to a woman at work who told me that women who get cervical cancer are promiscuous . . .' I was really angry. It can happen to anyone, not necessarily someone promiscuous. We are all at risk once we've had sex.

Also, I was put on the Pill when I was thirteen because of period problems. I keep wondering if that caused it. I didn't have sex until I was twenty-one, so it wasn't early sex . . . I used to smoke as well. But you may never do any of these things, and still get it.

[Support?] The service I had from doctors was good, because I asked for it. I'm confident, fluent and I want to know. We've got to encourage every woman to ask more.

My mother-in-law was great in the end, supportive and terribly worried.

I don't think my husband believed how serious it was; it was only when we heard about my having to have a hysterectomy that he really started to worry. If you ask friends, they would say I wasn't frightened, but with my husband, I'd get really morbid. There was a particular record that my husband bought . . . it will always be very special because it brings back memories of that period of my life, and wondering whether I'd be here the following Christmas.

I think in the end it was quite positive really. I've started doing things, writing leaflets, for the local Health Authority. Many women have said to me that they've found them helpful, and that's good. This all happened about five years ago. I know I'm fine now. I think I'm very lucky.

Evelyn

I wasn't due for a smear. I had one because I went to the Family Planning Clinic because I was taking a new lover.

229

I had a really good GP who, as soon as he heard, was on the phone to me straight away saying, 'Look my dear, it's important that you go and be seen to immediately. Don't hang about waiting for them. Just go.'

When I went for the examination, I was really impressed by the way the doctor gave time and attention and drew his little diagrams. He explained exactly what was happening and what they would do. It was good.

I had two or three smears, and then I went in for treatment. I had a cylinder biopsy, not a cone, where they take more cells away. I went in on a Tuesday morning and came out on a Friday. I don't really remember much about it. I remember coming out of the anaesthetic and Stanley (my husband) was there . . . then I woke up seemingly four hours later and Helen, my daughter, was there. They'd met in the corridor, so it must have been minutes in between!

Afterwards on the Friday, I went straight from the hospital to do a four-day workshop, and then went straight back to work on the Tuesday.

I don't know what caused it. I thought maybe that it was some kind of continual knocking through intercourse. I certainly haven't drawn any conclusions about numbers of partners. I don't think it could have been that.

At no time did I ever think it was cancer. I knew all the time that it wasn't. I knew from my mother and father that cancer 'is not our thing'. I knew then that none of us would die from that.

It played a very minimal part in my life really. There were a lot of other things going on for me at about the same time, and it just went into the melting pot.

[Support?] Well I did cry, but it's perfectly natural to feel upset. My lover wanted to come and see me in hospital, but we'd just split up, and I wouldn't let him. The doctor was very caring, and the hospital staff were good and at the right level for me, enough information and enough support. I got a lot of attention from people at work, and at the workshop I went to, and I got very close to my daughter when she came to see me in hospital.

It was really no sweat for me, though I think it was a big deal for other people.

Carole

For me, it started when I went for my regular smear. I had treatment for CIN 3 a few years ago, and so now I am on yearly tests just to make sure. I went for one just after Christmas, but at the time, I had some sort of mild infection that was causing a discharge, and the nurse warned me at the time that I'd probably have to come back for a repeat smear, as that might be clouding the result. Sure enough, about two weeks later I had a really nice phone call from my GP, saying that yes, they hadn't got a satisfactory result, and could I book in for another one in a month or two. I must admit, I kept forgetting; maybe some part of me knew something was wrong. In the end, I did book in, and almost immediately afterwards got another phone call from the doctor saying I had to go up for colposcopy.

I was halfway between upset and fine. I'd been through it all before, five years ago, and it was a bit traumatic. I suppose I'm lucky in that I've never worried about any of the 'sex stories' you hear – I know that isn't relevant to Patrick and me – so last time I simply had the treatment and got it over with. But whatever it was had come back, and that worried me.

231

My appointment was for a month's time, and at a different hospital from before, because we've moved house. In fact, everything was very different. I got a leaflet beforehand, with my appointment slip, telling me about the clinic, and also explaining that they often did treatment there and then, if it was necessary. That was a step forward.

On the day I did feel nervous, mainly in case they found that something had grown, something much worse than last time. The hospital waiting room was, I'm afraid, just as crowded as I remembered from last time, but they seemed to take a lot more care. I had a brief counselling session beforehand – unheard of in the 'old days' – and the nurse confirmed that I probably would be offered treatment the same day. That was fine by me.

Once in with the doctor, the routine was more or less the same: up on the couch, legs apart, the doctor taking a look. I loved watching the whole thing on a television monitor, though it seemed voyeuristic, somehow, even if it was my own insides! When the doctor eventually said that, yes, there seemed to be some problem, and yes I could have treatment there and then, I didn't actually hesitate, although I don't know what would have happened if I had said no – down off the couch and home in disgrace, I suppose! They gave me a local anaesthetic, which I have to admit hurt like hell, and then the treatment, which I didn't feel at all. I spent my time trying to answer the nurse as she made small talk to me. It must be really difficult for them, finding things to say to twenty patients a day in that situation.

When I got down off the couch I did feel shaky, and took the rest of the day off. Still, it was done, and it was actually nothing compared to the overnight stay I'd had last time. I

232

had to ring up in two weeks to find out if they'd got anything nasty from the biopsy, and this I did. No problem, all clear.

4 the resources

15 Resources section

Introduction

This section contains a list of resources which I or other women have found to be useful. They are arranged under subject heading—CIN/Cancer, Smoking etc. Where a resource is relevant to more than one heading, it has been listed more than once. This is to make it easier to use as a reference guide, but it does mean that if you read the text all the way through, it may get a little repetitive! Within each heading, I have listed leaflets, books, people to see, organizations and various other resources such as videos and tapes, so that you can easily find the type of resource you need. To save space, the organizations or contact points have usually been listed by name only and the full address and details are given in the separate address list at the end.

Remember that all details, including prices, may change with time, so it is often useful to check with an organization that their resources are still the same as when this book went to press.

It's noticeable that the majority of the organizations I have listed are in London or the South East. This is sad, but par for the course: nationwide organizations do often base themselves at the centre of communications. I have not been able to track down many support groups for CIN, so if you hear of one, do let me know. The provincial ones for cervical cancer are so numerous that it is probably worth your while approaching a national organization first and asking them for their local group.

Unfortunately, I have not had the opportunity to 'road test' all the resources mentioned here. The ones I have not seen, however, have been looked at by other women. Even so, mistakes do occur, or you may not receive the good service that others did. If you find a resource or organization to be unsatisfactory, do tell them and ask for improvement and, if you like, let me know too so that I can incorporate such information in future editions of this book.

Finally, I know I have not included all the resources that exist, because I do not know about everything in the field that is currently happening. So if you know of a good book, leaflet or support group that isn't mentioned here, please let me know.

CIN/Cancer

Leaflets

Many hospitals produce their own leaflets, and there are too many to mention here. Happily too, the number of leaflets produced by organizations has grown, and so here I offer a

simple listing of what is available. Most of them cover the
same ground, with perhaps a slight difference in emphasis
here and there.

An abnormal smear, what does that mean?, Women's Health,
40p plus sae.

Bodyimage, sexuality and cancer, Cancerlink, £1.75 (free if you
have cancer or are running a support group).

Calling all women, Women's Nationwide Cancer Control
Campaign, available in English, Gujerati, Punjabi, Bengali,
Urdu, Hindi, Turkish, Cantonese, Vietnamese, 15p plus p
and p.

Cervical cancer, the facts, Imperial Cancer Research Fund, free
in limited numbers.

Cervical cancer, Imperial Cancer Research Fund, free in
limited numbers.

Cervical smears, Marie Stopes House, available to clients
when you attend for diagnosis or treatment, or if you send
an sae.

Cervicography, Marie Stopes House, available to clients when
you attend for diagnosis or treatment, or if you send an sae.

Colposcopy, Marie Stopes House, available to clients when
you attend for diagnosis or treatment, or if you send an sae.

Life with cancer, Cancerlink, £2.75 (free if you have cancer or
are running a support group).

Women's cancers, something you can do, Imperial Cancer
Research Fund, free in limited numbers.

Leaflets suitable for distribution are available in packs of 100
for £2.00 plus VAT, p and p from Women's Nationwide
Cancer Control Campaign. Titles include: *Cervical smear
test; Why won't you have your smear test?; Have your mother
and grandmother had a smear test?; Have you been recalled for a*

239

smear test?; What is the wart virus?; Have you been referred to a colposcopy clinic?

Books

The Family Planning Association bookshop, at their main London office or by mail order, offers a full range of books and articles on cervical screening and cancer.

Barker, Graham, *Your cervical smear*, Adamson Books, 1987. This is a factual look at smear tests and what happens after them. You may find it useful to fill in more of the medical detail.

Chomet, Jane and Julian, *Smear test* Thorson's, 1991. This book is written, with her son, by the GP who bought a colposcope for her own surgery, to cut down waiting times.

Harvey, Judith, Mack, Sue and Wolfson, Julia, *Cervical cancer and how to stop worrying about it*, London, Faber & Faber, 1988 is also factual, but this time based around questions you might ask and concerns you may have.

Szarewski, Anne and Froog, Albert Singer, *Cervical smear test—what every woman should know*, Macdonald Optima, 1988. Written by two doctors experienced in cervical screening and treatment, this book gives an excellent breakdown of the issues involved.

People to talk to: one-to-one

There are many organizations offering counselling for all forms of cancer, including cervical cancer. Conversely, there seem to be no tailor-made counselling services for women with CIN, although all the general health organizations and most of the cancer organizations said they would be happy to help. Please note that some organizations and individual counsellors do charge a fee for their services, and you may want to check this ahead of time.

British Association for Counselling can recommend you to a one-to-one counsellor in your area. These counsellors will not usually specialize in medical problems, but can help you talk through your feelings about what is happening; normally counsellors charge fees for their work.

BACUP operates a one-to-one counselling service for cancer patients at their London offices, and are happy to talk about CIN conditions too.

The Bristol Cancer Centre is mainly a residential centre for teaching alternative approaches to cancer, but also provides free information and support on the telephone.

Brook Advisory Centres around the country provide free counselling to young people (under 25) on sexual issues including positive smears. You need to attend their clinic, and if they cannot help, they will refer you on. Contact them through their national office.

CancerLink has a telephone service which gives you information on cancer and CIN, and on the services they have available.

Cancer Relief provides home nursing and financial support for people with cancer and their families.

CYANA (Cancer–You Are Not Alone) offers a comprehensive service for all types of cancer. This includes one-to-one counselling for sufferers and their families and a 24-hour telephone service.

Positive Smear

Dr Jan de Winter Clinic for Cancer Prevention Advice aims to help you minimize the likelihood of contracting cancer, and supports cancer sufferers. It offers free counselling services on a one-to-one basis.

Marie Stopes Clinics is a private (i.e. fee paying) organization that provides a broad range of gynaecological services for women. They offer a telephone information service and helpline, plus hourly counselling for a fee.

New Approaches to Cancer offers a referral service for those wanting holistic treatment of all forms of cancer alongside their orthodox treatment. Their service is free, but the counsellor or therapist themselves may charge.

Tak Tent is a Scottish organization of support groups for cancer patients and their families. They also provide a one-to-one counselling service by people trained in counselling those with cancer.

Ulster Cancer Foundation offers telephone and free face-to-face counselling for all cancer sufferers and their supporters.

Women's Health (formerly the Women's Health and Reproductive Rights Information Centre) do not run a counselling service as such, but women are welcome to ring the health enquiry line to discuss any concerns or fears. They also have a database of women who are happy to share their experiences of cervical conditions. For contact details, ring the enquiry line.

The Women's Nationwide Cancer Control Campaign offers telephone counselling for all women with cancer, and has a sound knowledge of the problems involved in cervical cancer and CIN conditions. Their Helpline is open from 9.30am to 4.30pm Monday to Friday.

People to talk to: support groups

There are a number of support groups for cancer sufferers, though I could find none specifically for cervical cancer. At the time of going to press I could find few general ongoing support groups for women with positive smears. You could try going to an ongoing cancer support group, but may find that it does not deal only with cervical conditions. Also, there may be a 'mismatch' between your situation and the seriousness of the condition of some of the people in the group.

If you want to start a support group yourself for CIN or cancer sufferers, CancerLink offers support and training to those starting groups. *In Our Own Hands*, by Sheila Ernst and Lucy Goodison, published by The Women's Press, London, 1982 gives some useful guidelines for running groups.

The Bristol Cancer Centre has 110 support groups countrywide. Their structure varies, but all are free and all are based round the philosophy and approach of the Bristol Centre which teaches self-help and complementary therapies.

Cancerlink help people set up their own cancer support and self-help groups all over Great Britain and abroad. They have a Groups Support Service which acts as a resource, offering training information and support, publishes a quarterly newsletter and publishes a directory of support groups. They can put you in touch with a group or help you start your own. In particular, they have contacts with a network for lesbian women affected by cancer.

Cercan is a support group which was formed after a mix-up over smears in the Liverpool area resulted in some women being given a 'negative' result when in fact they had a positive condition. Some later developed more serious cervical conditions. Cercan is open to all women worried about a positive smear result. Contact Cercan via Liverpool Community Health Council, 57/59 Whitechapel, Liverpool L1 6DX, (051-236 1176).

CYANA (Cancer–You Are Not Alone) is a centre for sufferers of all types of cancer, which holds informal support group sessions weekly at their London Centre. A closed bereavement group counselling is also available.

New Approaches to Cancer is an umbrella for 300 support groups which are mostly free of charge and operate in varying ways, some once a week, some once a month, others on a drop-in basis.

Tak Tent runs nineteen support groups throughout Scotland. These are made up of patients, relatives and professionals involved in cancer care. They stress that these are support groups and professional-led, not self-help groups.

Tapes

The Bristol Cancer Centre offers a wide range of tapes about a complementary health care approach to cancer in general.

Videos

Most videos are not intended for personal or home viewing, but for support groups or medical professionals. Some suggest that you have a health visitor or nurse present to 'trouble-shoot' after the film, in case anyone is worried or distressed.

Cervical cancer is a video produced by Leicestersl
Authority which is relevant to CIN conditions as well as
cervical cancer. I have not seen it, but reports are good;
however I would suggest viewing it first before using it with a
group. Order from H. & H. Scientific Consultants, PO Box
MT27, Leeds LS17 8QP (0532 687189).

Cervical cancer–the facts from the Imperial Cancer Research Fund
is available from Plymouth Medical Films, Palace Vaults, 33
New Street, Barbican, Plymouth PL12 2NA (0752 267711). I
haven't been able to see or review this film, so you might like to
check its relevance to your group before buying it.

Down there is a video based on a play about women who have
had positive smears. It's funny, hard-hitting and feminist and
should be run with a discussion afterwards. It's available
from Albany Distribution, Douglas Way, London SE8 4AG
(071-692 6322).

Test in time is a video about smear tests prepared by and
available from the Women's Nationwide Cancer Control
Campaign. It shows what happens during the test and if any
abnormalities show up. It costs £25.00 to buy or £10.00 to
hire, both prices plus VAT and p and p, from WNCCC.

Thank you Doctor Papanicolou is a video of interviews with
women who have had experience of cervical cancer and with
health professionals. It challenges many of the
presuppositions and aims to help you work from a position of
strength. Available from Albany Distribution, Douglas Way,
London SE8 4AG (071-692 6322).

Telephone information lines

Healthcall provides a telephone service of recorded health

245

tapes. The numbers are: 0898 600732 (cervical cancer); 0898 600984 (cervical smears).

Other suggestions

The Cancer Relief Macmillan Fund funds Macmillan Nurses who give practical advice and emotional support to cancer patients and their families. It also provides financial support and day care centres.

The Imperial Cancer Research Fund is currently (1992) carrying out research into the effect that taking vitamin supplements and giving up smoking has on women with CIN 1. If you have this condition, and could travel to London once or twice in the course of the year to take part in the study, contact Dr Anne Szarewski or Sister Liz Upwood on 071-269 3006.

Hysterectomy

Leaflets

Many hospitals produce their own leaflets, and there are too many to mention here. Ask at your hospital or your Community Health Council for what is available.

Hysterectomy Support Group produces a leaflet *Hysterectomy, a new horizon,* price £1.25 plus sae.

Hysterectomy and vaginal repair is a leaflet written by Sally Haslett and Molly Jenkins who have both had hysterectomies. The leaflet covers practical aspects of preparing for and recovering from the operation. Send 75p to Box No. 1, St Thomas's Hospital, Lambeth Palace Road, London SE1 7EH.

Women's Health leaflet on *Hysterectomy* costs 40p plus sae.

People to talk to: one-to-one

The Hysterectomy Support Group was formed to encourage self-help through informal sharing of experience. This can be one-to-one, in telephone counselling or personal meetings. Several of the women I talked to mentioned this group and spoke positively about it. Contact person: Ann Webb.

Women's Health has a phone information service (see address list for hours of operation). It keeps a register of women who have had a hysterectomy and are willing to talk to others, and will refer to support groups throughout the country.

People to talk to: support groups

The Hysterectomy Support Group. This group has a variety of support groups for women and their partners. It meets in various parts of the country.

Telephone information lines

Healthcall provides a telephone service of recorded health tapes. The number is: 0898 600733.

Infections and viruses

Leaflets

All about warts and viruses, and *How to cope with thrush* are leaflets giving information on various relevant conditions. They are available from Women's Health, price 40p each plus sae.

People to talk to: one-to-one

The Herpes Association offers free counselling both by telephone and face-to-face to anyone troubled by herpes. *Women's Health* provides a telephone information and support service on a wide range of health issues including viruses.

People to talk to: support groups

The Herpes Association runs free support groups for members only; the times and locations are mailed to members every two months.

Telephone information line

Healthcall provides a telephone service of recorded health tapes. The numbers are 0898 600700 (genital herpes); 0898 600702 (other sexually transmitted diseases).

Contraception

Leaflets

The Family Planning Association has a number of short leaflets about all aspects of contraception. They are updated frequently, available in English and five Asian Languages and are all free if you send an sae. You will probably also be able to get them at your local Family Planning Clinic: *Your choices in contraception* (describing all methods); smaller leaflets covering the combined pill; the progesterone-only pill; IUD; diaphram, cp and sponge; natural methods; injectible methods; sterilization for men; sterilization for women; emergency contraception.

Women's Health provides several leaflets about contraception, prices ranging from 30p to 50p plus sae.

Books

There are a number of books on contraception, and it is difficult to recommend just one. The following have been mentioned to me as being particularly helpful by women I have spoken to.

The fertility and contraception book, Julia Moss and Josephine Heaton, Faber and Faber 1990. A practical book, but one which also looks at the emotional issues around choosing your method of contraception.

Safer sex–the guide for women today, Diane Richardson, Pandora Press, 1990. This AIDS-age book is a good, down-to-earth guide to safe sex and how to negotiate it, and

Positive Smear

put it into practice. It gives excellent coverage of all forms of barrier contraception.

The Family Planning Association bookshop, at their main London office or by mail order, offers a full range of books and articles on contraception.

People to talk to: one-to-one

Your local GP or Family Planning Clinic will usually be able to give you advice and support on methods of contraception, and on moving from one method to another.

Brook Advisory Centres around the country provide free counselling to young people (under 25) in sexual issues including contraception. You need to attend their clinic, and if they cannot help, they will refer you on. Contact them through their national office.

The Family Planning Association does not offer counselling, but if you contact their main office by phone or in person, they will give information and refer you on.

Women's Health offers a phone information and support service on a wide range of health issues including contraception.

Telephone information lines

Healthcall provides a telephone service of recorded health tapes. The numbers are 0898 600773 (barrier contraception); 0898 600938 (coming off the Pill); 0898 600625 (all methods of contraception).

General health

Leaflets

Women's Health provides a variety of leaflets about all aspects of women's health, including food, alcohol, housing and stress. For a full list write to them directly.

Books

Boston Women's Health Book Collective, *The new our bodies ourselves*, New York, Simon & Schuster, 1987. The new version of the old feminist favourite is even better than the original, with a comprehensive listing of all general health issues, and sections on issues particularly relevant to positive smears, cervical cancer, viruses and contraception.

People to talk to: one-to-one

Women's Health offers a phone information service (times given in address list) on a wide range of health issues. The phones are always answered by women, who understand women's problems and will do their best to advise and refer where necessary.

Telephone information lines

Healthcall provides a telephone service of recorded health tapes. The full directory, which contains over 420 different topics, can be obtained directly by ringing 0898 600600. Healthcall is not, however, a diagnostic service and cannot give you advice or counselling over the phone.

Smoking

Leaflets

ASH is a public information service that gathers and disseminates information on all aspects of smoking and which provides up-to-date information about how individuals can give up smoking. They can provide you with leaflets and other material to help you give up.

Books

Stop smoking, Penny Ross, Thorsons, November 1992; a new book, so I haven't seen this, but it deals particularly with one of the issues which may stop you smoking – the tendency if you do stop, to put on weight.

People to talk to: one-to-one

Women's Health offers a phone information and support service on a wide range of health issues, including smoking.

People to talk to: support groups

ASH provides workplace consultancy services which give advice and information to companies on introducing a no-smoking policy.

Telephone information lines

Healthcall provides a telephone service of recorded health tapes. The numbers are 0898 600875 (women and smoking); 0898 600726 (how to stop smoking).

Complementary medicine

Leaflets

The Bristol Cancer Centre produces a number of leaflets on complementary approaches to cancer care, including some on its special diet, relaxation and meditation, and Bach Flower Remedies. A full list of leaflets and their prices can be obtained by contacting BCC direct.

New approaches to cancer. A leaflet on alternative and holistic approaches to cancer is available if you send them an sae.

Alternative medicine: promoting good health is a leaflet about the alternatives to orthodox approaches. It is available from Women's Health, price 40p plus sae.

Books

There are many books on complementary medicine.

New Approaches to Cancer and *The Bristol Cancer Centre* both offer a selection of books on holistic approaches to cancer. They will send you a list on receipt of an sae.

Boston Women's Health Book Collective, *The New Our Bodies Ourselves*, New York, Simon & Schuster, 1987. Has a comprehensive listing of all general health issues, often with an alternative slant.

People to talk to: one-to-one

The Bristol Cancer Centre is mainly a residential centre for teaching alternative approaches to cancer. It also provides free information and support on the telephone.

The Institute of Complementary Medicine will refer you to counsellors and alternative practitioners who can give support.

The Matthew Manning Centre offers one-to-one healing sessions with Matthew Manning himself.

New Approaches to Cancer offers telephone counselling and free face-to-face counselling to those local to Surrey.

Women's Health offers a phone information and support service on a wide range of health issues and will advise you on complementary medicine if they can.

People to talk to: support groups

The Bristol Cancer Centre has 110 support groups nationwide. Their structure varies, but all are free and all are based round

the philosophy and approach of the Bristol Centre which teaches self-help and complementary therapies.
New Approaches to Cancer helps form local support groups based around the principles of complementary medicine.

Tapes

The Bristol Cancer Centre offers a wide range of tapes about a complementary health care approach to cancer in general.
The Matthew Manning Centre has a series of audio tapes; write to the centre for a full list and prices.

Telephone information services

Healthcall provides a telephone service of recorded health tapes. The number is 0898 600897 (new approaches to cancer).

Other resources

Organizations

BUPA offers a course for nurses in cervical screening, which includes training in counselling.
The Cancer Research Campaign gives grants for research into, among others, all aspects of cervical cancer and screening including the psychological and emotional aspects.

Positive Smear

Community Health Councils. Your local CHC will usually be able to put you in touch with local support groups, health information services and pressure groups. If you have problems with medical practitioners, they will also support you in obtaining your rights. Find them in your phone book or Yellow Pages.

The Health Education Authority provides lists of publications relevant to a whole variety of medical subjects including cancer, available on request.

Marie Curie Cancer Care offers nationwide screening training for nurses, which includes coverage of the emotional and psychological aspects of supporting patients. They are always happy to look at setting up courses in areas that do not already have one.

The Myrtle Peach Trust is a registered charity that raises money for cervical cancer, principally within Milton Keynes, but ultimately for research which will help nationwide.

Books

The Best Counselling Guide, Susan Quilliam and Ian Grove-Stephensen, Thorsons 1991. This is a consumer guide to counselling, outlining how to get and keep the counselling relationship you want; it also contains an up-to-date comprehensive listing of all main counselling organizations in Great Britain.

I'm alive, Lily Hopkins, Changing Places Publications 1990: an account of Lily's work, centred around her campaign against the misdiagnosis of smear tests in Liverpool.

Women's Health have a large library of resources which includes books on cervical cancer and all other relevant topics, and is open to the public 11am-5pm Monday, Wednesday, Thursday and Friday.

Taking a helping hand by Jane Faulkwhynes is an account of her experiences at the Bristol Cancer Help Centre after a positive smear diagnosis. It is available from the Help Centre, price £3.75 plus p and p.

Address list

ASH (Action on Smoking and Health) 109 Gloucester Place, London W1H 3PH (071-935 3519).

Association for Neuro-Linguistic Programming, 48 Corser Street, Stourbridge, West Midlands DY8 2DQ. (0384 443935).

BACUP (British Association of Cancer United Patients and their Families and Friends), 3 Bath Place, London EC2 (Freephone 0800 181199 for information service; for other calls, new phone number imminent so ring Directory Enquiries)–10am-7pm Mon-Thur, 1pm-5.30pm Friday, then answering machine service outside these hours.

Bristol Cancer Help Centre, Grove House, Cornwallis Grove, Clifton, Bristol BS 4PG (0272 743216; 08.45am-1.45pm Mon-Fri, then answering machine).

British Association for Counselling, 1 Regent Place, Rugby, Warwickshire CV21 2PJ (0788 578328, 08.45am-5pm Mon to Fri, then answering machine).

Brook Advisory Centres, 153a East Street, London SE17 2SD (071-708 1234; Mon-Thur, 9am-5pm, Friday 9am-4.30pm, then answering machine).

BUPA Health Screening Centre, Battle Bridge House, 300 Gray's Inn Road, London WC1X 8DU (071-837 6484).

Cancerlink, 17 Britannia Street, London WC1X 9JN (071-833 2451; Mon to Fri 9.30am-5pm plus answering machine [client line]; 031-228 5557; Mon to Fri 10am-5pm plus answering machine [client line]).

Cancer Relief Macmillan Fund, 15-19 Britten Street, London SW3 3TZ (071-351 7811).

Cancer Research Campaign, 2 Carlton House Terrace, London SW1Y 5AR (071-930 8972 (office)).

Community Health Councils can be found in your local phone book or Yellow Pages.

Co-counselling Phoenix, 5 Victoria Road, Sheffield S10 2DJ (0742 686371).

CYANA (Cancer–You Are Not Alone), 31 Church Road, London E12 6AD (081-553 5366; Mon to Fri 9am-4.30pm plus answering machine).

The Family Planning Association, 27-35 Mortimer Street (071-636 7866; Mon to Fri 10am-3pm).

Health Education Authority, Hamilton House, Mabledon Place, London WC1H 9TX (071-383 3833).

The Herpes Association, 41 North Road, London N7 9DP (Helpline number 071-609 9061, available twenty-four hours a day).

The Hysterectomy Support Network, 3 Lynne Close, Green Street Green, Orpington BR6 6BS (081-856 3881 [message on where and how to obtain information about hysterectomy]).

Imperial Cancer Research Fund, PO Box 123m, Lincoln's Inn Fields, London WC2A 3PX (071-242 0200; 9am-5.30pm).

Institute of Complementary Medicine, PO Box 1941, London SE16 1QZ (071-237 5165; 9am-4.30pm then answering machine).

The Irish Family Planning Association, 36-37 Lower Ormond Quay, Dublin 1, Republic of Ireland (Dublin 725366 and 725394).

The Dr Jan de Winter Clinic for Cancer Prevention Advice, 6 New Road, Brighton, Sussex BN1 1UF (0273 727213).

Marie Curie Cancer Care, 11 Lyndhurst Gardens, London NW3 5NS (071-435 4305; 9am-5.30pm [enquiries only]).

Marie Stopes House, 108 Whitfield Street, London W1P 6BE (071-388 8090 [advice line]; 071-388 0662 office hours plus answering machine); 10 Queen Square, Leeds (0532 440685 office hours plus answering machine); 1 Plice Street, Manchester (061-832 4260 office hours plus answering machine).

The Matthew Manning Centre, The Green, Hartest, Bury St Edmonds, IP29 4DH (0284 830222 [direct line for general information]).

Myrtle Peach Trust, (Mrs Maureen Pruskin, Fund Co-ordinator/Press Officer), Laser and Colposcopy Clinic, Milton Keynes Hospital, Eaglestone, Milton Keynes MK6 5LD (0908 660033, x. 2830).

New Approaches to Cancer, 5 Larksfield, Egham, Surrey TW20 0RB (0784 433610).

Plymouth Medical Films, Palace Vaults, 33 New Street, Barbican, Plymouth PL1 2NA (0752 267711).

Tak Tent, Cancer Support Scotland, G Block, Western Infirmary, Glasgow G11 6NT (041-334 6699 and 041-357 4519; 9am–2pm then answering machine).

Ulster Cancer Foundation, 40-42 Eglantine Avenue, Belfast, BT9 6DX (0232 663439; 9.30am-12.30pm weekdays, 2pm-4pm Wednesday [care information service], 0232 663281 9am-5pm plus answering machine [office]).

Women's Health (formerly Women's Health and Reproductive Rights Information Centre), 52 Featherstone Street, London EC1Y 8RT (071-251 6580; 11am-5pm Mon, Wed, Thur, Fri).

Women's Nationwide Cancer Control Campaign, Suna House, 128-130 Curtain Road, London EC2A 3AR (071-729 4688).

16   Questions to ask

This is a summary of the questions you could ask your doctor or consultant at various stages of your diagnosis and treatment. They are all given at appropriate places in the book, but I have gathered them together here for easy reference.

Questions to ask your GP or Family Planning Clinic if you see them after your positive smear:

> What is my smear test result?
> What severity of condition have I got?
> Is there any other evidence to indicate what my condition is?
> Is there any sign of infection? A virus?
> Do I need to see a consultant? When? Where?
> How will the appointment be made?

Is there any chance that I will be offered treatment immediately after the examination (*See and Treat*)?
Do I need to come back to you for a repeat smear? When?
Should I make the appointment now?

Questions to ask your consultant when you go for further examination:

What is your name? What sort of doctor are you? What job do you do in the hospital?
What is the nurse's name? Will she stay in the room with me?
What has my GP said to you in his letter?
Are you going to do another smear? A colposcopy? A punch biopsy?
Will there be anyone else in the room while I'm being examined?

Questions to ask your consultant after a colposcopy/punch biopsy, or at diagnosis stage:

What has my GP/clinic said to you in the letter?
Are you going to take another smear? Photograph of my cervix? Colposcopy? Biopsy?
Will I have the opportunity for treatment now if your examination suggests that is possible?
What exactly did you find during your examination?
What was my repeat smear/cervicography result?
What did the biopsy show?
What grade of CIN do I have?
How far has it spread?

Can you tell me now whether my condition is cancerous or pre-cancerous?

Questions to ask your doctor or consultant about inflammations, infections or viruses:

Did you notice any inflammation on my cervix? Do you know what might be causing this?
Was there any vaginal discharge? Can you suggest what might be causing this?
Did you find any evidence of infection or viruses?

Questions to ask your consultant concerning the treatment s/he suggests:

Do you think I need treatment? If not, why not?
What treatment do you think would be best for me?
Why are you choosing this sort of treatment?
When will this treatment happen? Now? How long will I have to wait?
What will be the after effects of this treatment (on my ability to have children, make love, etc)?
Will my treatment mean my changing methods of contraception (will I have to have my IUD removed)?
What would be the position if I wanted to have . . . (any other form of treatment than the one the doctor has mentioned)?
Why would you not recommend this?
I am concerned about these things; could I talk them through with you?
Will I be an out-patient? (If so, when, for how long?)
Will I be an in-patient? (If so, when, for how long?)

Last words

Towards the end of each interview I asked all the women this question: 'What do you want to say to the people who read this book?' This is what they replied:

It's a problem that concerns women; it's not caused by women. (Diana)

Keep going, everything is going to be OK. Don't feel dirty, or guilty. Don't panic. Fight for what's best for you. (Heather)

The operation is only a day of pain; it can be got rid of. (Rachel)

Cheer up. It's not that bad. You're getting through it. (Janet)

Take notice. Women should get together. (Emma)

In the last resort, I wasn't just a cervix. I didn't have to do what I was told. (Jane)

Loads of people have it, loads of people have to go through it . . . no problem. (Jo)

Just keep asking the questions . . . just keep pushing. (Rosemary)

Make sure you get looked after. (Evelyn)

Look! It happened to me and I'm OK! (Jane B.)

Notes

1. See letter from David Hicks and Valerie Brown, Jessop Hospital for Women, Sheffield, as written to *The Lancet* 4 March, 1989.
2. Richardson, A.C. and Lyon, J.B., 'The Effect of Condom Use on Squamous Cell Cervical Intrapithelial Neoplasia', *American Journal of Obstetrics and Gynaecology*, vol. 140, No. 8, (1981), 909ff.
3. Harris, R.W.C., *et al*, 'Characteristics of Women with Dysplasia or Carcinoma in Situ of the Cervix', *British Journal of Cancer*, vol. 42, (1982), 359.
4. Dr Peter Skrabenek, as reported in the *Irish Medical Times*, 14 March 1986.
5. McCormick, J.S., 'Cervical Smears, A Questionable Practice', in *The Lancet*, 22 July, 1989, p.207.
6. Skrabanek, P., Cervical Cancer Screening, Update in Women and Health, 15 April 1990.
7. As reported in *The Age*, October 1991.
8. Saveria Campo M., Vaccination against Papillomavirus, *Cancer Cells*, Vol. 3, No.11, p.421, November 1991.
9. Cuzick, J. *et al*, 'Human papillomavirus type 16 DNA in cervical smears as predictor of high-grade cervical cancer', *The Lancet* Vol. 339, p.959, April 1992.
10. Anderson, M.C., *et al*, *A Text and Atlas of Integrated Colposcopy*, (Chapman and Hall, 1992).
11. Robinson, Jean, 'Cancer of the Cervix: Occupational Risks of Husbands and Wives and possible Preventative Strategies', in *Pre-Clinical Neoplasia of the Cervix, Proceedings of the Ninth Study Group of the Royal College of Obstetricians and Gynaecologists*, Jordan, J.A. and Sharp, F., and Singer, A. (eds), (Royal College of Obstetricians and Gynaecologists: London 1982), pp.11-27.

12. McAvoy, B.R. and Raza, R. – 'Asian Women, Contraceptive Knowledge, attitudes and usage, Contraceptive services and cervical cytology', *Health Trends* 1988, No. 1 Vol. 20 11-17.
13. These theories are based on a number of studies carried out over the past twenty years, as reported in most basic gynaecological textbooks, eg Boon Mathilde E, and Tabbours-Boumeester, Meete-Lise, *Gynaecological Cytology* (London, Macmillan, 1980).
14. Turner, M.J., *et al*, 'The male factor in cervical neoplasia', *Contemp Rev Obstet Gynaecology* Vol. 1 September 1988.
15. See correspondence in *The Lancet*, 25 April 1987, McCance, D.H., Human Papilloma Virus and Cervical Cancer.
16. Tidy, J., *et al*, 'High Rate of Human Papillomavirus Type 16 Infection in cytologically normal cervixes', *The Lancet*, 25 February 1989.
17. Meanwell, C.A., *et al*, 'HPV-16 DNA in Normal and Malignant Cervical Epithelium: Implications for the Aetiology and Behaviour of Cervical Neoplasia', *The Lancet*, 28 March 1987. See also the editorial of the same issue, 'the case against the papilloma virus is far from proven'.
18. Wickenden, C., *et al* 'Prevalence of HPV, DNA and viral copy numbers in cervical scrapes from women with normal and abnormal cervices', *Journal of Pathology*, vol. 153 (1987) 127-35.
19. Murdoch, J.B., Cordiner, J.W. and MacNab, J.C.M., 'Relevance of HPV-16 to laser therapy for cervical lesions', *The Lancet*, 20 June 1987.

20. Murdoch, J.B., *et al*, 'Histological and cytological evidence of virus infection and human papillomavirus type 16 DNA sequences in cervical intrapithelial neoplasia and normal tissue in the west of Scotland; evaluation of treatment policy'.
21. Gagnon, F., 'Contribution to the Study of the Etiology and Prevention of Cancer of the Cervix and of the Uterus', *American Journal of Obstetrics and Gynaecology*, vol. 60, (1950), 516.
22. Skrabanek, P., 'Cervical Cancer in Nuns and Prostitutes, a plea for scientific continence', *J Clin Epidemiology*, Vol. 41, No. 6, pp.577-582, 1988.
23. *Positive Smear, A Positive Approach*, Conference Report.
24. Mack, S., *et al*, *Positive Smear Update Report* 1991.
25. As reported in *The Guardian*, 28 November 1990.
26. Wiseman, A.: 'A pilot study on information manipulation on patients in the Colposcopy Clinic, 1987-8'.

General references

27. Doherty, I., *et al*, 'The assessment of the psychological effects of an abnormal cervical smear result and subsequent medical procedures', *Journal of Psychosom. Obstet. Gynaecol* March 1992, pp.319-324.
28. Boag, F., *et al*, 'Assessment of psychiatric morbidity in patients attending a colposcopy clinic situated in a genitourinary medicine clinic' *Genitourinary Med* 1991; vol. 67, 481-484.

Index

270

272